DUAL DIAGNOSIS WORKBOOK

by Dennis C. Daley, MSW

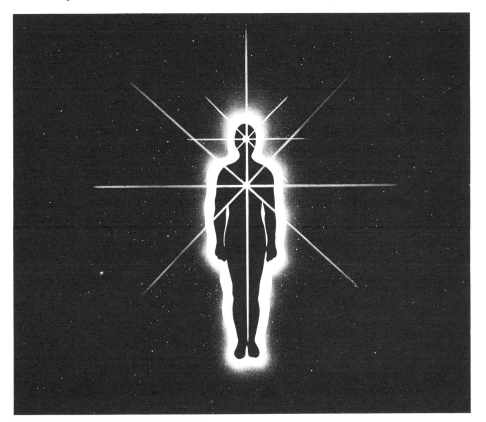

Recovery Strategies for Addiction and Mental Health Problems

Foreword by Terence T. Gorski

Herald House / Independence Press
Independence, Missouri

Acknowledgments

I wish to thank the many patients in our dual diagnosis programs who gave me ideas on topics to include in this workbook. Thanks to my colleagues in the dual disorders programs at Western Psychiatric Institute and Clinic, University of Pittsburgh Medical Center, for their support and interest in using my recovery materials in patient and family education programs. I also wish to thank Terence T. Gorski for his helpful feedback on this workbook, and to Jim Hough of Herald Publishing House. And a very special thanks to Cindy Hurney for her outstanding skills in word processing. Cindy helped to make this more attractive and "user friendly," and her competence is most appreciated.

Additional copies of this workbook are available from the publisher:
　　　Herald House/Independence Press
　　　3225 South Noland Road
　　　P.O. Box 1770
　　　Independence, MO 64055-0770
　　　Phone: 1-800-767-8181 or 816/252-5010

Copyright ©1994
Dennis C. Daley, M.S.W.

ISBN 0-8309-0666-5

Item # 17-024670

Table of Contents

Foreword

Dual diagnosis, the treatment of patients who have chemical dependency and other mental and personality disorders, is a growing problem in the behavioral health care field. It is estimated that 40–70 percent of all mental health and chemical dependency clients are actually suffering from dual disorders.

The current treatment delivery systems are designed to treat either chemically dependent patients or mental health patients. There are very few dual diagnosis programs that have a staff trained in both chemical dependency treatment and the treatment of other mental health disorders. To further complicate the situation, the mental health field and the chemical dependency field use a different language to deliver services they provide. The conceptual differences between these two fields often makes it difficult to provide an integrated treatment plan.

I have known Dennis Daley for more than fifteen years. I have been impressed by the extensive work he has done in dual diagnosis. Dennis has been "down in the trenches" with chemically dependent people who have mental and personality disorders for years. He has taken a highly scientific and critical approach to developing treatment for dual disorder patients. All of his methods have been field tested where it counts — in individual and group therapy sessions with some of the most difficult dual diagnosis patients you can find.

The *Dual Diagnosis Workbook* presents proven strategies that can and do work for dual diagnosis patients. As I reviewed the manuscript I was impressed with the clear, concise, and simple terms in which everything was described. I can envision clinicians using this workbook directly with dual diagnosis patients. More importantly, I can see that these techniques, if used as designed, will work to produce sobriety and emotional stability in patients.

The provision of dual diagnosis treatment requires a basic understanding of chemical dependency, Axis I Mental Disorders, and Axis II Personality Disorders. The interaction between chemical dependency, mental disorders, and personality disorders also has to be understood. These differences need to be overcome in an operationalized treatment plan.

Dennis Daley has integrated chemical dependency and behavioral health treatment in a unique way, focusing on didactic group therapy using structured sessions. He provides topic-oriented discussions, brief educational interventions, and individual treatment planning principles. He also provides outstanding resources in the form of a bibliography and suggested reading to guide clinicians to a more in-depth understanding of the procedures they are working with.

I believe this *Dual Diagnosis Workbook* is a major contribution to the field of chemical dependency and mental health treatment.

Terence T. Gorski

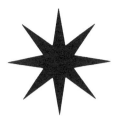

SECTION I

Understanding Dual Disorders
and
Recovery

SESSION 1

How to Use This Recovery Workbook

This recovery workbook was put together for several reasons:

1. to give you information about psychiatric disorders and alcohol/drug abuse (a condition referred to as "dual disorders");
2. to give you information about the recovery process from dual disorders;
3. to help you take an active role in taking steps to get well and cope with your disorders and problems contributing to them or resulting from them; and
4. to help you identify specific recovery and relapse prevention issues to focus on in a systematic way.

This workbook was developed as a result of discussions with many patients who gave their input on topics to include in it. Many felt one comprehensive workbook made it easier to complete and keep track of recovery assignments. If you want additional information on any of the topics discussed in this workbook or in group sessions, talk with your therapist or other treatment team member. Together you can decide on other readings or assignments to help you reach your goals while you are in treatment.

In this workbook you will find information on the issues that other clients with dual disorders felt were the most important ones to focus on in treatment. These issues include:
- understanding mental health and addictive disorders
- identifying why you came to treatment and setting goals
- working through denial and overcoming roadblocks to recovery
- understanding the recovery process from dual disorders
- effects of dual disorders
- coping with feelings such as anger, anxiety, boredom, and depression
- changing behaviors, personality, and thinking
- developing your spirituality
- developing structure and a daily plan of recovery
- improving family and personal relationships
- coping with social pressures to use alcohol or drugs or stop taking medications
- building a support system or recovery network
- making lifestyle changes
- the importance of follow-up treatment after participation in hospital-based or residential treatment
- using AA/NA/CA, mental health support groups, and recovery clubs
- developing a relapse prevention plan
- having an emergency plan

Everyone needs to go at their own pace in recovery. Therefore, do not rush through this workbook. Take things slowly and focus on one or two changes at a time. Sometimes it helps to work on one section and "test out" new ideas before going on to the next section. You can use this workbook over a very long period of time.

Be as honest as you can when you work in this guide. Discuss your struggles or difficulties with your therapist.

The sections you work on will depend on your special problems and needs as well as the length of time you are in treatment. It is recommended that you discuss completed sections with a member of your treatment team or sponsor. They can give you valuable feedback and guide you on choosing which sections to work on.

This workbook was designed to help you develop your personal recovery plan. Be realistic when you set your goals for change. Accept even small steps as a sign of improvement. Don't get down on yourself if you make a mistake or have a setback. Just keep working your recovery plan and things will get better. It is your responsibility to read and finish assignments. It requires you to take an active role in your treatment. You have a big say in getting well and making positive changes. Change is hard, but you can do it. Just keep trying. Also, make sure you keep all of your scheduled treatment appointments with your therapist or doctor. If you want to stop treatment or feel upset, angry, or frustrated with your treatment, talk it over with your therapist. Together you can figure out what's going on to make you feel this way.

I developed this workbook from many years working with people who have psychiatric disorders, addiction, or both. I believe the topics covered include the ones that people with dual disorders are most concerned with and need to address in their ongoing recovery. Some of the workbook activities are adapted from my other writings. Other activities are new. All have the same basic purpose—to help you help yourself in recovering from dual disorders and improve the quality of your life.

SESSION 2
Understanding Mental Health and Addictive Disorders

The National Institute of Mental Health conducted a major study of adults in the United States to determine how many had a mental health or alcohol/drug problem at some point in their lives. The results of this large study showed:

- More than 22 percent of adults either currently or in the past have had a mental health problem.
- More than 16 percent of adults either currently or in the past have had an alcohol or drug problem.
- 29 percent of people who experienced a mental health problem also had an alcohol or drug problem at some time in their lives.
- 37 percent of people who experienced an alcohol problem also had a mental health problem at some time in their lives.
- 53 percent of people who experienced other types of drug problems (cocaine, marijuana, opiates, etc.) also had a mental health problem at some point in their lives.

Many other studies of people seeking care for psychiatric disorders or seeking care for an alcohol or drug problem have been conducted. These studies also show that many people have more than one disorder. In fact, some people have two or more different types of psychiatric illness in addition to an alcohol or drug problem.

These studies show that alcoholism and other drug dependencies are very common among adults. These diseases often accompany mental health disorders, causing much suffering for the affected individual as well as the family.

Because alcohol and drug addictions affect mental health problems and recovery from them, and because mental health disorders affect the use of alcohol or other drugs or recovery from addiction, treatment must address both disorders together. Focusing on recovery from only one of your disorders (your addiction or mental health disorder) puts you at risk to relapse to the other. Therefore, recovery must address both of your disorders.

To recover you must develop a specific plan to learn how to stop using alcohol or other drugs and to remain abstinent once you stop. Your plan must also address your coexisting psychiatric disorder. Recovery means not only addressing your specific disorders but learning to live a healthy and balanced lifestyle. This requires you to learn new, healthy ways of thinking, managing your feelings, relating to other people, and coping with your problems and symptoms. Put simply, recovery is about positive change in yourself and your lifestyle.

Understanding Alcohol and Drug Addiction

A number of different types of legal and illegal chemicals are used and abused by people with concurrent psychiatric disorders. These include alcohol, marijuana, crack or cocaine,

10

other stimulants, opiates such as heroin, tranquilizers, PCP, hallucinogens, and inhalants. Despite all the current focus on drugs such as crack cocaine, the number-one drug of abuse remains alcohol. In fact, many more people die each year or experience serious medical or life problems from alcohol than cocaine or other street drugs.

While street drugs such as crack cocaine, heroin, or marijuana are abused by many people with psychiatric disorders, so are prescribed drugs such as tranquilizers or pain medications. Many people get hooked on prescription drugs they initially took for medical or psychiatric symptoms. Some of these people exhibit a lot of "drug-seeking" behaviors. They go from doctor to doctor to get drugs for a variety of complaints or symptoms such as anxiety or sleep difficulties. As soon as they think a particular drug isn't helpful, they increase the amount they take of this drug. Or they seek other types of medications. The result is that they become addicted to prescription drugs.

Addiction, similar to other diseases or illnesses, has a cluster of symptoms. According to the American Psychiatric Association, you meet the criteria for alcohol or drug dependence if you have three or more of the following symptoms:
- excessive or inappropriate use of alcohol or drugs;
- preoccupation with getting or using alcohol or drugs;
- a significant increase or decrease in your tolerance to alcohol or drugs;
- experiencing withdrawal symptoms once you stop completely or cut down your use of alcohol or drugs;
- using alcohol or drugs to avoid withdrawal sickness;
- having trouble cutting down or stopping once you drink or take drugs;
- quitting for a period of time only to go back to using again;
- continuing to use alcohol or drugs despite the fact that such use causes you problems;
- experiencing problems in one or more areas of your life as a result of your use of alcohol or drugs; or
- giving up important activities due to your alcohol or drug use.

If you have fewer than three of these symptoms and your life is harmed in some way as a result of your use, your condition is referred to as "substance abuse." A big mistake many people make is believing they have to be "physically addicted" to alcohol or drugs or use almost every day in order to qualify for having an addiction. *Nothing could be further from the truth.* Many people who don't use every day and who don't show every symptom listed above still have a serious problem with alcohol or other drugs. Therefore, keep in mind that either "substance abuse or dependency" can cause much heartache and suffering and interfere with recovery from psychiatric illness. Sections 4 and 5 of this workbook will help you further examine your specific experience with alcohol and other drugs. An excellent resource in this field is *Learning to Live Again: A Guide for Recovery from Chemical Dependency* by Merlene Miller, Terence T. Gorski, and David Miller.

Acute and Chronic or Persistent Psychiatric Illness

Some people have only one or two *acute* episodes of a psychiatric illness during their lifetime. They may not experience their illness throughout their lives. Other people have *recurrent* psychiatric illness and experience three or more episodes throughout their lives. Many experience some symptoms continuously over time. This is called *chronic or persistent* psychiatric illness. This type is usually more disabling and often requires long-term care under the direction of a psychiatrist or psychologist. However, many people with chronic psychiatric illness have periods when they do very well and their symptoms remain under control.

Types of Psychiatric and Addictive Illness

There are many different types of illnesses among adults. They show in symptoms related to your moods, thoughts, behaviors, and ability to function in daily life. The most common categories of psychiatric illness found among people who have drug or alcohol use disorders include the following:

1. Mood Disorders. These include serious disturbances in your mood or how you feel. The most common is *major depression,* which involves feeling sad or blue, loss or decrease in interest in life, difficulty concentrating, appetite or sleep problems, decline in energy, feelings of guilt and worthlessness, and thoughts about whether or not life is worth living. These symptoms are present most of the time, nearly every day for two weeks or longer.

Another type of mood disorder is called *recurrent depression.* This condition refers to having three or more different episodes of depression over time. Months or years may separate the episodes of depression. *Seasonal depression* refers to episodes of depression that tend to occur during specific times of the year such as during the winter. *Dysthymia* refers to a more chronic type of depression in which symptoms are more or less experienced for a long time, often two years or longer. In some cases of depression, suicide is planned or even attempted. Drinking alcohol or taking other drugs can raise the risk of suicide because chemicals either impair judgment or give the person courage to try suicide.

Some people switch back and forth between depression and mania, while others experience just one of these mood disorders. People who have both types of mood disorders have *bipolar disease* or *manic-depressive illness.* Some even experience symptoms of both depression and mania at the same time, a condition referred to as *bipolar disease, mixed.*

Mania is the opposite of depression in that the mood is very high instead of low. Energy and activity levels increase and the need for sleep decreases. The person is easily distracted and their thoughts may race. During a conversation, they may jump from topic to topic. Because their judgment is affected, they may do foolish things, go on spending sprees, put themselves in danger, or get involved in a lot of activities at once.

Drugs and alcohol are often abused during the time when the person's mood is elevated. Patients sometimes talk about missing the "high mood" associated with bipolar disorder and may use cocaine or other stimulant drugs to recapture that "high" feeling.

2. Anxiety Disorders. These are characterized by worrying too much, feeling a sense of dread, or feeling very anxious. These disorders usually include both physical and mental symptoms that affect the person's life in one or more ways.

Symptoms of anxiety may also be present in other psychiatric disorders such as depression. Many people get hooked on alcohol or drugs like tranquilizers as a way of reducing their anxiety symptoms. In the long-run, however, things get worse because an addiction develops.

A *phobia* is an irrational fear of a situation or object so strong that it causes distress and problems in the person's life. *Social phobias* involve irrational and intense fears of being looked at, criticized or rejected by others, or acting in ways that will be embarrassing or humiliating. Some people have many social situations they are afraid of while others have only one or two situations they fear. The more common social phobias include dating; speaking, writing, or eating in public; or taking tests. *Simple phobias* involve irrational fears of situations such as being in a closed space, being in a high place, traveling by bus or plane, or fears of objects such as bugs, snakes, blood, or needles. One type of phobia, called *agoraphobia*, often makes the person a prisoner at home due to the fear of leaving. The person with agoraphobia may never or seldom leave home as a result. A phobia usually is not based on reality and causes the person to avoid the situation or object that is feared.

Panic disorder involves sudden attacks in which the person feels an intense and overwhelming feeling of terror. The person may worry about going crazy, dying, or feel that things "don't seem real." The person may feel dizzy or faint, shake or tremble, sweat, feel sick to the stomach, experience hot or cold flashes, or even feel chest pains or a racing heart.

Obsessive-compulsive disorder involves repeating behaviors like hand washing, checking doors, windows, or the stove, or counting objects many times. The person often believes bad things will happen if these rituals are not repeated a certain number of times. This disorder also involves the recurrence of obsessions or senseless and frightening thoughts, over and over again.

Generalized anxiety disorder involves more or less continuous, unrealistic, and excessive anxiety and worry about two or more areas of life. This anxiety and worry is accompanied by other symptoms such as trembling; feeling shaky, dizzy, restless, hyper, keyed up, or on edge; shortness of breath; increased heart rate; nausea; hot flashes or chills; trouble concentrating or "going blank"; and irritability.

Post-traumatic stress disorder (PTSD) refers to the development of symptoms that follow a psychologically upsetting event such as combat, torture, a serious threat to one's life or that of family or close friends, rape, or destruction of one's home or community as a result of a disaster. This event comes back in the form of recurrent dreams or thoughts about it or feeling like it is happening again. Seeing things that are a reminder of the event can also cause severe distress. People with PTSD avoid things associated with the trauma or feel "numb" about it and detach from others as a result. Other symptoms of PTSD include trouble sleeping or concentrating, angry outbursts, or being hypervigilant.

Alcohol and tranquilizers are commonly abused by people with various anxiety disorders. These chemicals help decrease anxiety symptoms at first, but they often lead to dependency.

3. Schizophrenic Disorders. This category of mental illness is characterized by disturbances in the thought process. People suffering from *schizophrenia* have trouble telling the difference between reality and fantasy. The capacity to respond emotionally is also affected, and they may become withdrawn or unpredictable. People with this type of illness may hear voices or have beliefs that don't make sense such as "Others are out to get me" or "They put thoughts in my mind." Some exhibit strange or unusual behaviors like talking to themselves in public or dressing in a very bizarre manner.

4. Personality Disorders. These disorders involve ingrained personality traits that show in a person's behaviors, leading to serious problems in life or a great deal of personal distress. These problems are usually repeated throughout life because the personality traits are so entrenched and hard to change.

There are many different types of personality disorders. Each involves a number of specific personality traits involving self-defeating behaviors that together cause the person to feel a great deal of personal distress and/or have trouble getting along at work, school, home, or with others. Some problematic traits and behaviors associated with personality disorders include: strong mistrust of people, emotional coldness and aloofness, extreme self-centeredness, being overly dramatic, needing constant attention and admiration, lacking empathy or concern for others, being dishonest and lying, cheating or deceiving others, being unconcerned with the laws or rules of society, extreme shyness, impulsivity (acting before thinking), and excessive dependency.

5. Other Addictive or Compulsive Disorders. These involve compulsive gambling, overeating, or sexual activity that is "out of control." The individual is unable to stop these behaviors despite the fact that they are causing problems. Oftentimes the family may be aware of the problem but denial prevents the individual from seeing the addiction or asking for help. Many people have more than one type of addictive disorder. And many also have other psychiatric conditions such as depressive illness or a personality disorder.

Dual Disorders (Psychiatric Illness and Alcohol/Drug Abuse)

As I mentioned before, many people with psychiatric illness also have an alcohol or drug problem, a condition referred to as *dual disorders*. Having a psychiatric illness increases the risk for an alcohol or drug problem. Likewise, having an alcohol or drug problem increases the risk of psychiatric illness.

Alcohol and drug abuse sometimes makes existing psychiatric symptoms worse or causes new symptoms. For example, some patients end up in the psychiatric hospital after abusing drugs like cocaine, marijuana, or alcohol and becoming severely depressed, manic, psychotic, or suicidal. In some cases the use of these substances made patients stop taking medication for their psychiatric illness or stop counseling sessions. In other cases, alcohol or drug use made the medications for the psychiatric illness less effective or ineffective. If you take an antidepressant or antipsychotic medicine while using alcohol or other drugs, it can raise or lower the level of medicine in your blood, thus altering its effectiveness. Your medicine just won't work like it should if you drink alcohol or take street drugs or other nonprescribed drugs.

Some people develop an alcohol or drug addiction before experiencing a psychiatric disorder. Others develop their addiction after an expisode of psychiatric illness. Regardless of which of your disorders came first, you still have to address both. Otherwise, you won't recover.

> *"Addiction and mental health disorders are coexisting diseases that usually need to be treated together for recovery to progress."*

Causes of Psychiatric Illness and Addiction

There is no one simple way to explain why you developed a psychiatric illness or addictive illness. Try to accept your illnesses as "no fault" caused by a combination of factors working together. No one "chooses" to have bipolar illness, schizophrenia, alcoholism, cocaine addiction, or other disorders. Medical and social scientists who study psychiatric illness and addictive illness tell us that they may result from these factors:

1. Biological. Many illnesses such as depression, bipolar disease, schizophrenia, and alcoholism run in families. Scientists believe that some of us inherit a "predisposition" to develop certain illnesses. There may be something in our brain chemistry or other biological aspect of our bodies that makes us predisposed to having an illness. Just as diabetes, hypertension, or other medical problems run in many families, so too do psychiatric and chemical addiction disorders. In other words, heredity stacks the deck against some of us.

The acute and long-term effects of alcohol and drugs can also cause psychiatric symptoms. Medical and health problems contribute to psychiatric disorders as well.

2. Psychological. Our beliefs about the world and ourselves, how we think, our personality, the ways we cope with stress and problems, and how we act may impact on whether or not we experience a psychiatric illness. Some of us react differently to ordinary life stresses or problems than others. This means that some people are more psychologically vulnerable than others.

3. Environment. Our family, community, living environment, and culture affect us as well. Any of these factors may in one way or another impact on psychiatric illness or addiction. Some people are more apt to abuse alcohol or drugs or develop psychiatric problems as a result of these or other environmental factors.

A formula that simplifies the many complex factors that contribute to psychiatric illness and addiction is illustrated in the charts below.

Biology + Psychology + Environment

+ Stress = Psychiatric Illness

Biology + Psychology + Environment + Stress

+ Alcohol/Drugs = Addiction

The Importance of a Good Assessment

Because the effects of alcohol and drugs can mimic, cover-up, trigger, or exaggerate any psychiatric symptom, you may need to be off alcohol and drugs for a couple weeks or longer before an accurate diagnosis can be given. You can help the assessment process by being totally honest about your symptoms and your alcohol and drug use patterns.

A good assessment usually involves one or more interviews with health care professionals who ask you questions about different psychiatric symptoms, alcohol and drug use, your medical history, and your personal and family history. Your assessment may also involve a physical examination and lab tests or urinalysis tests to determine what drugs are in your system or whether there are medical conditions caused by alcohol or drug use. Psychological tests may be used as well. Your assessment may involve filling out "self-reports" or questionnaires. While in some cases assessment goes fairly smoothly, in other cases it is quite complex, difficult, and takes time. Make sure you find out your diagnoses from the professionals who evaluate you.

The more you understand your diagnoses, the more you will understand how treatment can help you and what steps you can take to help yourself. You may be asked to involve your family or significant others in assessment and treatment. They can provide useful information to your treatment team. And they may be a source of help and support to you. Treatment involvement can help families understand their own feelings and reactions as well. Sometimes other family members may be in need of their own treatment for a psychiatric or addiction problem. Of course, it is ultimately up to you whether or not to involve your family or other significant people in your treatment. If you have reservations about involving others in your treatment, discuss these with your treatment team.

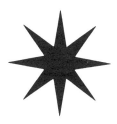

SECTION II

Setting the Foundation
for
Recovery

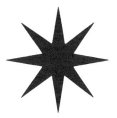

SESSION 3
Why I Came to Treatment

One of the first important tasks of recovery is to identify the symptoms and problems that led you to treatment for your dual disorders. In early recovery the focus is mainly on stabilizing your symptoms and figuring out your longer-term recovery plan. Following is a brief list of some of the more common symptoms of psychiatric disorders and addiction that cause people to come to a treatment program. Put a √ next to the problems and symptoms below that you think played a role in your coming to treatment, regardless of whether you came voluntarily or not.

____ depression

____ manic behavior or very high moods

____ self-harm (cutting or burning self, overdosing on pills, etc.)

____ violence toward others

____ suicidal thoughts, plans, or attempt

____ severe agitation

____ severe anxiety

____ severe panic attacks

____ obsessive thoughts

____ compulsive rituals (counting, checking, etc.)

____ sexual problems

____ hearing voices

____ having paranoid, unusual, or very strange thoughts

____ alcohol abuse or addiction

____ crack/cocaine abuse or addiction

____ other drug abuse (heroin, pot, pills, hallucinogens, PCP, etc.)

____ compulsive gambling

____ compulsive overeating

____ compulsive sexual behavior

____ serious problems with spouse, partner, or other family member

____ serious problems with roommates or friends

____ unable to take care of myself

____ quit taking medication and got sick

_____ bad temper problems

_____ in trouble with the law

_____ had no place to live

_____ ran out of money

_____ involuntarily committed to treatment

_____ pressured by family to get help

_____ pressured by the legal system (parole/probation) or a social service agency to get help

Identify any other psychiatric or personal problems that contributed to the need for you to be in treatment at this time:

_____

_____

_____

_____

_____

Describe what you think caused your psychiatric disorder:

_____

_____

_____

_____

_____

Describe what you think caused your alcohol and drug problem:

_____

_____

_____

_____

_____

Anthony's Reasons for Coming to the Hospital

I was doing real good for awhile. Then I missed some counseling sessions and ran out of my antidepressants. Since I was feeling pretty good, I just quit my treatment altogether. In a few weeks I got real down. I couldn't shake it and began drinking and using drugs again. Told myself some alcohol and herb would lift my spirits. All it did was make me worse. Got more depressed. When I went back to the crack pipe, didn't care what happened to me. Wasn't important if I lived or died. That's how desperate I felt before coming to the hospital. I know now I gotta get back on track. Get clean and stay clean, and stay in treatment for my depression.

Kim's Reasons for Seeking Outpatient Treatment

I can't seem to stay away from the alcohol. I get a few weeks sober then drink again. I feel nervous and depressed almost all of the time and can't get rid of my obsessive thoughts. I know this sometimes leads me to drinking because the longer I'm off alcohol, the worse I feel. And, my relationships are the pits. For some reason, I drive my friends away. They tell me I'm too intense and demanding. I don't know how to have a good relationship and always hook up with the wrong kind of guy. I need help with a lot of things, not just my drinking. Therapy helped me in the past. I hope it can help me again.

SESSION 4
My Alcohol and Drug History

The first step in getting clean or sober is admitting that you have a problem with alcohol or other drugs. One of the ways you can do this is to take a close look at your alcohol and drug use and how it has affected your life. Answer the following questions about your alcohol and drug use. Share your answers with a counselor; an AA, NA, or CA sponsor; or other trusted person.

1. I've used alcohol, street drugs, or nonprescribed drugs in the past as follows (fill in number of times):

	90 Days	Year	In My Lifetime
Alcohol			
Marijuana or Hash			
Cocaine or Crack			
Opiates or Narcotics			
Tranquilizers or Downers			
Stimulants or Uppers			
PCP or Angel Dust			
Hallucinogens or Acid			
Inhalants: Glues, Aerosols, etc.			
Other drugs (Write in)			

2. I've gotten high on drugs or alcohol too many times to count.

____ *Yes* ____ *No*

3. I've experienced the following symptoms or behaviors in relation to alcohol or drug use (✓ the items that apply):

____ *Excessive or inappropriate use of alcohol or other drugs:* getting high or drunk and not being able to fulfill my obligations at home, work, or with others; feeling like I need chemicals to fit in with others or to function at work or home; driving under the influence of alcohol or drugs; using alcohol to help me come down off drugs; using drugs so I can drink more alcohol or party longer; overdosing on drugs.

_____ *Preoccupation with getting or using chemicals:* living mainly to get high on alcohol or drugs; being obsessed with using; hiding or protecting my supply of alcohol or drugs.

_____ *Changes in tolerance:* needing more alcohol or drugs to get high; getting high much easier or with less alcohol or drugs than in the past.

_____ *Having trouble cutting down or stopping once I drink or take drugs:* not being able to control how much or how often I use; using more alcohol or drugs than I planned.

_____ *Withdrawal symptoms:* getting physically sick when I cut down or stop using (for example, having the shakes, feeling nauseous, having gooseflesh, having a runny nose, or other types of "jonesing"); experiencing mental symptoms such as depression, anxiety, or agitation.

_____ *Using alcohol or drugs to avoid or stop withdrawal symptoms:* using chemicals constantly to avoid withdrawal sickness; drinking or using drugs to stop oncoming withdrawal symptoms; drinking in the morning to stop the shakes.

_____ *Getting into trouble because of alcohol or drug use:* losing jobs or being unable to find a job; getting arrested or having other legal problems; losing relationships or having trouble with family or friends; or money problems.

_____ *Continuing to use alcohol or other drugs even though they cause me problems:* ignoring the advice of my doctor, therapist, or other professional to stop using because of the problems that chemicals have caused me; using again even though I know such use causes me medical, emotional, family, work, legal, financial, or spiritual problems.

_____ *Giving up important activities or losing friendships because of my use:* stopping activities that once were important to me; giving up friends who don't get high; losing friends because of the way my alcohol and drug use affects my behavior with others.

_____ *Stopping my use for a period of time (days, weeks, or months), only to go back again:* staying sober or clean for awhile, then justifying a return to alcohol or drug use.

_____ *Blackouts:* forgetting what I did or said while under the influence of alcohol or other drugs.

4. Write in the number of addiction symptoms you checked off: _____

If you checked three or more symptoms, you have a dependency problem. If you checked one or two, you still have a problem that will interfere with your psychiatric recovery if you don't do something about it.

5. Which of the following high-risk behaviors have you participated in related to your alcohol or drug use? Place a ✓ next to the ones you have experienced.

____   Shooting drugs with a needle

____   Sharing needles, cotton, or rinsing water with others, or using unsterile needles

____   Smoking crack, or freebase cocaine

____   Overdosing on drugs

____   Going to "shooting galleries" or "crack houses" to get high

____   Lying to doctors, nurses, or dentists in order to get drugs

____   Going to a hospital emergency room and faking symptoms to get drugs

____   Trading sex for alcohol or drugs, or to get money for chemicals

____   Drinking mouthwash or other products for the alcohol content

____   Committing crimes to get money for alcohol or drugs

____   Getting arrested as a result of using (DUI, public intoxication, etc).

6. On a scale of one to ten, how would you rate your problem with alcohol or drugs?

1	3	5	7	10
Somewhat of a problem	Moderate Problem	Serious Problem	Very Serious	Severe or Life threatening
_____	_____	_____	_____	_____

7. On a scale of one to ten, how would you rate your need for treatment for your alcohol or other drug problem?

1	3	5	7	10
No need for treatment	*Some need for treatment*	*Moderate need for treatment*	*Great need for treatment*	*Extreme need for treatment*

_____   _____   _____   _____   _____

8. From reviewing my completed checklist I would say this about my alcohol and drug use:

_____

_____

_____

Leroy's Review

After thinking about my alcohol and drug use, I'd have to say my addiction has kicked my ass real good. I been getting high on booze and dope a long time, too many years to count really. OD'ed couple a times, lied, cheated, scammed, stole, lost jobs ... you name it, I did it. If I couldn't get dope, I'd drink. Ain't no doubt about it, my addiction is bad. Been a big factor in going to jail and going in and out of detox centers and psychiatric hospitals.

Gail's Review

Until recently, I never really considered myself an addict because I didn't use street drugs. All I used was alcohol and pills that I got from doctors. Many, many pills. Got them from a couple of doctors at the same time. The thing is, I lied about my symptoms so that I could get the pills I thought I needed. Since they were for my back pain and my nervousness, and doctors gave me them, I didn't think I had an addiction problem. When I look at how many pills I'd been using and what I'd do to get them, there's no doubt that I'm an addict. I know the reason I never made much progress with my psychiatric problem before was that I kept using pills that I shouldn't have been taking. Plus, I kept lying over and over, to my doctors, my therapist and to myself. To recover I know I have to be honest about this because my way hasn't got me anywhere but in trouble. I can't go through my life taking a pill every time I'm upset, have pain or have some other symptom.

SESSION 5
Effects of Dual Disorders on My Life

Addiction, psychiatric illness, and dual disorders can affect any area of your life. This includes your physical health; your relationships with family, friends, and coworkers; your ability to take care of your basic needs; and your overall adjustment and happiness. An important part of early recovery is taking a look at the effects of your dual disorders on your life. Although this can cause you some anxiety at first, it can help motivate you to work hard at your recovery.

In your own words, state how you think your disorders affected different areas of your life. There may be an overlap in some of these areas.

	Psychiatric Illness	Alcohol or Drug Use
Physical Health (including medical and dental problems)		
Diet and Eating Habits		
Sexual Desire or Behavior		
Exercise Habits		
Self-esteem or Confidence		
Relationships with Parents		
Relationships with Spouse or Partner		
Relationships with Children or Stepchildren		
Relationships with Boss or Co-workers		

	Psychiatric Illness	Alcohol or Drug Use
Relationships with Friends		
Spirituality (relationship with God or Higher Power, religious practices, etc.)		
Work or School		
Lost Opportunities or Wasted Talents or Abilities		
Hobbies, Leisure Interests, or Recreational Practices		
Financial Condition		
Difficulty with the Law or Other Legal Problems		
Other Problems		

In reviewing my answers I would say this about how my dual disorders have affected my life:

Sandra's Review

Both my problems really messed me up. My depression, cutting myself, and getting into fights got me in trouble with the law. Plus it made my kids real upset. Almost got busted and sent to jail. When I was at my worst, I thought about overdosing on dope to end it all. I just didn't have nothing to live for.

When I was shooting drugs, I didn't care who I got high with. It's a wonder I didn't get AIDS 'cause I shared needles. It even got worse when I started smoking crack. I traded sex for drugs and got hooked up with some nasty dudes. But to get the rocks, I'd do any damn thing.

Drugs caused me to lose a couple jobs. Then, I quit caring whether I worked or not. It didn't matter. My kids are real important but when you doin dope, don't nothing matter as much as getting high. Got so bad I couldn't take care of them. Children and Youth Services was in my face and I almost lost my kids.

You could say my life's been messed up real bad by what I done. Made me feel like I was a nobody. Man, I guess I'm lucky I ain't dead or nothing, or in jail. Least now I got a chance to get myself together.

SESSION 6
My Problem List and My Strengths

List below the specific problems you need to work on first while in treatment. These should relate to the reasons you sought help on your own or were committed to treatment. This list should include both your psychiatric and your alcohol/drug abuse disorders.

1.   *Psychiatric*

_____

_____

_____

2.   *Alcohol/Drug Abuse*

_____

_____

_____

3.   *Family or Relationship*

_____

_____

_____

4.   *Other (legal, work, living arrangements, etc.)*

_____

_____

_____

Russell's Problem List

I know I have a lot of problems to work on, but these are the ones I have to focus on when I'm in the hospital:

1.   Feeling depressed and not caring about anything in my life or having any goals or direction.

2.   Crack, alcohol, and marijuana abuse.

3.   I was living with other addicts who still get high. I need to find a sober/clean living environment.

4.   I got a short fuse and need to learn how to control my anger and rage 'cause it gets me in fights.

Juanita's Problem List

I want to get myself together and work on these problems with my doctor and outpatient therapist:

1.   Being impulsive and dropping out of treatment as soon as I feel better or when I get upset with my counselor.

2.   Alcohol and drug abuse and how it put a wedge between me and my children.

3.   I'm a real nervous person and worry all the time. I need to learn to cope with my nervousness without getting high.

4.   I have trouble keeping a job. I either miss a lot of work and get fired or quit 'cause I don't like my boss.

My Strengths

It is helpful in recovery to build on your strengths. Your strengths refer to things that are positive about yourself or your life. They include:

- Your positive qualities such as being kind, assertive, creative, hardworking, or open and honest with others.

- Your attitudes and motivation such as really wanting to stay clean and make things better in life, being committed to recovery, or wanting to get ahead in life.

31

- Your lifestyle such as having a job, adequate money to take care of your needs, leisure interests and hobbies you enjoy, and goals you are working toward.

- Your religious or spiritual beliefs or believing that you are capable of getting better.

- Your relationships such as having family or friends you are close with and who support and care about you.

List three or more strengths or positive aspects of yourself, your life, or your relationships:

_____

_____

_____

_____

_____

_____

_____

Shawna's Strengths

1. *I'm a good mother to my children and like taking care of them. I give them lots of love and attention.*

2. *I don't give up easily. I work hard to get ahead and don't give up when things get rough.*

3. *I have a good sense of humor. My friends think I'm pretty funny.*

4. *I'm really motivated to change. I want to stay clean and get my life together. I want to quit doing things to hurt myself and others.*

5. *I don't mind asking others for help. I'm willing to let my NA sponsor and treatment team help me.*

SESSION 7
My Goals While I'm in Treatment

Choose two problems from your list in Session 6 that you want to work on now. Describe each of these problems, then list your goal(s) and steps you can take to help you achieve these goals while you are in treatment. If you aren't sure what to work on first, ask your doctor or therapist to help you. The problems and goals that you work on will change during the course of your treatment. Start working on your most pressing problems first.

Problem 1 - Psychiatric (Brief Description)

_____

_____

My *Goal(s)* in relation to this problem:

(1) _____

_____

(2) _____

_____

***Steps* I can take to reach my goal(s):**

(1) _____

_____

(2) _____

_____

(3) _____

_____

(4) _____

_____

(5) _____

_____

Problem 2 - Alcohol or Drug Abuse (Brief Description)

_____

_____

My *Goal(s)* in relation to this problem:

(1) _____

_____

(2) _____

_____

Steps I can take to reach my goal(s):

(1) _____

_____

(2) _____

_____

(3) _____

_____

(4) _____

_____

(5) _____

_____

SESSION 8
Advantages of Recovery

Giving up alcohol and drugs and getting involved in recovery from dual disorders takes hard work. It may be difficult at first to imagine what it will be like to give up chemicals.

List the advantages and disadvantages of giving up alcohol and drugs:

Advantages	Disadvantages

List the advantages and disadvantages of staying involved in dual recovery:

Advantages	Disadvantages

Good-bye Letter

Imagine you could say anything you wanted to your addiction in a good-bye letter. In the space that follows, write a letter to your addiction, expressing all your feelings about what addiction has done to you and what it will be like to live without chemicals.

Dear Addiction:

_____

_____

_____

_____

_____

_____

_____

_____

_____

_____

_____

_____

_____

_____

_____

_____

SESSION 9
Medical and Psychiatric Effects of Drugs and Alcohol

Drug and alcohol use can cause medical and mental health problems. Chemical dependency puts you at a higher risk for medical problems such as liver disease or AIDS. Existing problems can worsen or new problems may develop due to:

- The direct effects of chemicals on your body
- Accidents caused by being under the influence of chemicals
- Your diet and health care habits
- Impurities in drugs
- Complications caused by mixing drugs or using drugs and alcohol together
- Complications caused by using dirty needles to inject drugs, snorting, or smoking drugs
- Engaging in high-risk behaviors (for example, unprotected sex)
- Your overall lifestyle

In addition, alcohol and drugs can cause, worsen, or mask psychiatric symptoms, or they can contribute to relapse. Alcohol and drugs often interfere with recovery from psychiatric illness.

Answer the following questions regarding the effects of alcohol and drug use on your medical or psychiatric health:

1.   As a result of my alcohol/drug use, I've experienced:
         ____   An injury from an accident (home, work, car, boat, etc.)
         ____   Anxiety, confusion, or depression
         ____   Blackouts (periods of time I can't remember)
         ____   Close to death experience
         ____   Dental cavities or loss of teeth
         ____   Diet problems (poor diet, don't follow special diet, etc.)
         ____   Digestive system complications (ulcer, gastritis, pancreatitis)
         ____   Emotional turmoil
         ____   Frequent headaches, bouts with the flu, or generally feeling sick
         ____   Frequent visits to doctors, clinics, hospitals, or emergency rooms
         ____   Hearing voices (hallucinations)
         ____   Heart pain, heart attack, heart muscle damage
         ____   Hepatitis

_____ HIV-positive or AIDS

_____ Liver disease

_____ Lung disease or damage

_____ Nosebleeds

_____ Overdose of drugs

_____ Poor eating habits

_____ Poor health care habits

_____ Psychiatric problems

_____ Seizures or convulsions

_____ Sexual problems (difficulty performing, loss of interest in sex)

_____ Weight gain or loss of ten pounds or more (unintentional)

_____ Withdrawal sickness when I cut down or stopped using chemicals

_____ Worsening of other medical or psychiatric conditions (diabetes, depression, etc.)

2. Other problems I've experienced that are not included in the preceding list are:

_____

_____

_____

_____

3. The last time I had a physical examination was:

_____

4. The last time I had a dental examination was:

_____

5. I exercise:

_____

6. One *goal* related to my physical or mental health that I would like to work on is:

_____

_____

Potential benefits of reaching this goal are:

_____

_____

When I reach this goal, I will reward myself by:

_____

_____

Richard's Goal

I used to be a great athlete until drugs got the best of me, causing me medical problems. Lost a lot of weight and became run-down. My first goal is to get my health back. I can do this by staying off drugs and not drinking alcohol since booze always leads me back to drugs. Been fooling myself too long about the alcohol. I'm also following a routine now so I can get enough rest and sleep at night. Going to bed by midnight and getting up by eight so I get started for the day. I'm eating decent meals at regular times. Plus, I'm working out four times a week to help me get back in shape. I need this discipline to get my health and my self-respect back.

SECTION III

Accepting Your Disorders
and
Developing a Recovery Plan

SESSION 10

Denial in Addiction and Psychiatric Illness

This was written to help you understand what denial is, how it's related to your chemical dependency and psychiatric illness, and why it's critical to work through it in order to recover.

Try to relate the material and stories to your life as much as possible. Talk about your questions, concerns, and reactions with your therapist, other helping professional, or an AA/NA sponsor.

Listen to what Lamont, Karen, Bill, and Lisa say about their chemical use or psychiatric problems. See what you can learn about denial from them.

Ain't Nobody's Business What I Do

All my running people get high. It's the thing to do. Ain't no big thing, really, getting high on crack. Don't do it every day. You'd do it too if you lived in my neighborhood. It really ain't nobody's business what I do. What I do is on me and I'm telling you man, I like to get high.

Yeah, I got busted by the cops. But hey, they had it in for me. Got a bad break, that's all. My PO makes me go to these damn meetings and get slips signed. Gotta go to counseling too and piss in a bottle. He don't know nothing 'cause he ain't never been where I am. Talking about me being an addict just because I smoke some rocks. — **Lamont, age 27**

I Like to Get High

OK, so I like to get high. I've been getting high since I was fourteen. I enjoy getting loaded. Taking drugs makes me relax and feel mellow. I'm a real nervous type of person, but drugs help calm me down. I don't use needles or "hard" stuff like heroin or cocaine. Believe me, there's a lot of people worse off than me.

I don't think that drugs affect my work. I have a job and hardly ever miss work. In fact, I just got a raise. I don't ever use when I visit my parents and they've never seen me loaded. And drugs don't affect my relationships. Most of my friends like to get high, too. I'm not hurting anyone else. I have a right to get high if I want to. If drugs really get out of hand, then I'll probably quit. But for now, I just don't want to stop. — **Karen, age 34**

What's So Wrong with Feeling So Good?

I've always been an energetic person. I like working a lot and being involved in life. I can't help it if I don't need much sleep and get up early in the morning. What's wrong with being on the go all the time and wanting to accomplish things? Everyone is so negative these days. I want to be a positive person and get things done. You can't sleep your whole life away. It's a drag when you're not active and it gets real boring. There's just so much to do.

My wife and sponsor think I need to see a shrink. What the hell do they know about me? I think they're jealous because I feel so good and accomplish so much. They need to take their own inventory and not mine, and stay the hell out of my business. What's so wrong with feeling so good, like you can do anything at all? After all, I'm making lots of extra money because I can work so many hours. Besides, I like feeling on top of the world. And why in the hell should my wife get on me for spending money. After all, I'm making good money so why can't I spend a few hundred here and there. My wife is upset because I bought some golf clubs. I've always wanted to play golf, so what's the big damn deal? My wife is also upset because I bought some stock with the kids' college money. Hey, I found some good stocks and I know I'll make a killing and probably triple their money.

These people keep bugging me, especially my wife. She also accuses me of snapping out at her and the kids and being unreasonable. What can I say? If the kids mess up, I'm just going to tell them and get on them to clean up their acts. What's so unreasonable about this. Can't a father discipline his kids without his wife butting in? She should talk, because I've heard her get on the kids many times.

I'm just going to keep on doing what I've been doing. Work hard, stay active, and look for opportunities to make money. I know I can make a bundle. Everyone wants to get rich, don't they?   — Bill, age 42

I Should Be Able to Pull Myself Up

I've been clean from dope for almost eight months now and don't understand why I'm depressed. There's no reason why I shouldn't be able to pull myself out of this. My therapist and doctor want me to take medications for depression. But I kicked a big dope habit and have been clean eight months. I used every day for a couple of years. If I can kick my heroin addiction, there's no reason why I can't shake my depression. I want to be totally clean and off all drugs. I'll just keep working and pull myself out of this. After all, I'm a strong woman. I think if you can stop shooting dope, you should be able to do anything.   — Lisa, age 29

Many people like Lamont, Karen, Bill, and Lisa experience problems because of their drinking or drug use, their psychiatric illness, or both. Yet many outright deny their alcohol or drug use is a problem or that they have a psychiatric disorder. Some even deny both disorders. Why do they do this?

Denial is a refusal to believe or accept some painful reality in our lives. It's a "defense mechanism" that occurs without our being aware of it. It happens unconsciously and "protects" us from anxiety that comes from facing the truth about having a serious problem such as an addiction or psychiatric disorder.

Denial is what prevents people with alcoholism or other drug dependency from seeking help. It is considered the "fatal aspect" of the disease of chemical dependency because the end result of untreated addiction may be an early death or some other very serious consequence. Denial also prevents many people with psychiatric disorders from seeking help. As a result, many continue to suffer with their symptoms or continue to act in ways that interfere with their well-being or happiness. Some only get help as a result of an involuntary commitment.

Examples of Denial

Your denial may show in many ways. You may deny your psychiatric illness, your addiction, or both. Some people deny one of their disorders by blaming all their problems on the other. As you review the following list of some of the ways denial shows, make a note of the ones you relate to.

- Not believing you have a problem with alcohol or drug use despite evidence to the contrary.

- Minimizing your alcohol and drug use and believing "It's not that bad." After all, others use more stuff or more often than you.

- Blaming difficulties on "other" problems (boss, spouse, friends, pressures, mental illness, etc.) and not your substance use.

- Admitting to a problem with alcohol or drugs but refusing to do anything about it.

- Believing you can "cut down" and limit how much or how often you use, especially if you get help with your psychiatric disorder.

- Believing that because you are giving up your main drug of abuse, you can still use other chemicals (for example, giving up crack but drinking alcohol or smoking pot).

- Thinking that because you don't use large quantities, don't use every day, or don't get loaded every time that you use, you can't have a serious drug or alcohol problem.

- Thinking you can't be hooked because you don't suffer physical withdrawal symptoms when you stop using, or don't always "crave" alcohol or drugs.

- Believing after a period of sobriety and recovery that your problem is "under control" and you can handle a few drinks (pills, tokes, lines, etc.).

- Saying that you can't have a problem because you hold a job, take care of your family, haven't gotten into major difficulties, or don't act "crazy."

- Believing that no one else has been affected by your drinking or other drug use, or your psychiatric problems.

- Blaming your psychiatric symptoms and problems on your use of alcohol or other drugs.

- Believing that if you stop using alcohol or drugs, your psychiatric problems will be taken care of.

- Believing that because you are a strong person, you surely can't have a psychiatric disorder.

- Blaming your psychiatric problems on bad luck, bad breaks, or bad friends.

The cases cited earlier show different examples of denial in relation to addiction and psychiatric disorders. Lamont got busted by the cops and was forced to go to NA meetings and counseling, but he didn't think smoking crack was a problem. Karen denied she had a problem because she didn't use "hard stuff" like heroin or cocaine and didn't think her drug use affected her life in any negative ways. In fact, Karen saw drugs as "helping" her because it reduced her anxiety. Bill did not admit that anything was wrong with him despite the fact that his manic behavior became increasingly worse. And Lisa minimized her depression, particularly because she felt she should be able to "pull herself up."

To other people, denial of addiction may come across as willful lying or conning. They usually see your situation more clearly than you do because your judgment is impaired by your substance use, or you have blackouts and don't remember being loaded or the things you said or did while under the influence. Denial of your psychiatric disorder may come across to others as poor judgment on your part. They may wonder why you can't see that you have a psychiatric problem. Your illness itself can contribute to denial.

Family and Societal Denial

Family members can deny or minimize the effects of either or both of your dual disorders. They may not want to believe or accept the reality that you are an alcoholic or drug addict, or have a psychiatric illness. It may bring too much shame or embarrassment on them. With dual disorders some families may blame all of your troubles on your addiction and refuse to accept that you also have a psychiatric disorder. Or they may accept that you have a psychiatric illness and deny that your alcohol or drug use has anything to do with your difficulties.

The Effects of Denial

Many people with dual disorders never get help or don't get the correct help because of their denial. As a result, they experience negative consequences. The following comments show different effects of denial of addiction, psychiatric disorders, or both:

- *Everybody knew I was messed up on crack. Everybody but me, that is. I stole, lied, conned, scammed, cheated, and ripped people off to get money for some rocks. It was an everyday thing. My woman left me and told me she didn't want nothing to do with me unless I stopped getting high. Even my momma told me to straighten myself out and get off the crack 'cause it was messing with my mind. Got popped by my PO for violating my probation, but I still didn't think my drug use was that bad. Crack made me lose everything, even my freedom, before I saw it as my addiction.* — **Tony, age 26**

- *For years I prescribed myself a lot of different drugs to feel better and control my anxiety. Then I started using cocaine. Even though things got real bad, I still used drugs. After all, I'm a doctor and know what's best for me. I continued to deny my drug addiction until I lost my license to practice medicine. My husband left me and my life was shattered. I felt guilty, shameful, and very depressed. My life had no meaning. It took awhile, but I finally rebounded and put my life back together. But only after I got help for both my addiction and depression.* — **Ruth, age 35**

- *For years, everyone knew I was an alcoholic. Yet I continued to deny it. I drank heavily my whole life. It messed up my family and my health. Some friends ditched me because of how I acted. It wasn't until I suffered with gastritis and my doctor convinced me to get help that I stopped drinking.* — **Matt, age 57**

- *After I got hooked on heroin and cocaine, I lost my business, sold all of my assets, and spent more than $100,000. I got so desperate that I resorted to selling drugs to support my addiction. I ended up getting arrested a couple of times. It was after I lost my dignity that I got very depressed and even thought of killing myself. It wasn't until I got busted by my PO and spent some time in jail that I came to my senses. After jail, I went to a treatment program and NA.* — **Bill, age 31**

- *I quit or lost a lot of jobs because my panic and anxiety symptoms caused me to miss a lot of work. I became undependable. I lied to cover my tracks, but this didn't work. I often told myself I was getting bad breaks, that this was the reason for my job problems. Until I accepted that I had a mental problem and got help I wasn't able to break this pattern.   — Cindy, age 41*

- *I lost my daddy to drugs. He told us to quit bugging him about drugs, that he had things under control. He just wouldn't stop. I really miss him. Why did he have to die from taking drugs?   — Lara, age 12*

- *My wife and daughter kept telling me that I needed help when my mood became real high, but I ignored them. As my mania got worse, I did crazier things. I really hurt my family and put my job in jeopardy. But I was lucky and finally got forced to get help before I lost everything.   — Ron, age 39*

- *I've always had psychiatric problems and had no trouble admitting these. But addiction? No way. I used alcohol and drugs to have fun, calm me down, or make my hallucinations go away for awhile. Then I'd usually stop taking my medication, which always led to my getting sicker. A couple times I ended up back in the psych hospital. It was only after I finally admitted to my addiction that I started to get better. Since being straight for more than nine months, my schizophrenia isn't as bad.   — Rebecca, age 21*

- *I was a con long before I got hooked on booze and drugs. I stole, cheated, lied, and took advantage of everyone I could. Used women for whatever I could get from them. Wasn't nobody important to me, and I only looked out for number one. Sold drugs and stolen property to support my lifestyle. I lived on the edge and got in a lot of fights. Got shot once and stabbed a couple times. Messed up too many people to count. Spent time in prison twice and mental institutions too many times to count. Wasn't until I quit blaming society for my troubles and made a decision to get clean and stop this craziness that things changed. My problems messed me up for a lot of years.*
  — Carlton, age 29

These brief quotes show a variety of effects of denial. Many medical, emotional, social, family, financial, legal, and spiritual problems are caused by denying one or both of your dual disorders.

Why Deny Your Addiction or Psychiatric Problem?

The actual effects of alcohol or other drugs can contribute to your denial. For example, you may feel good after drinking alcohol, feel energized after snorting cocaine or smoking crack, or feel mellow after smoking pot or taking an opiate drug. Chemicals may even make your psychiatric symptoms better. After all, how can something that feels good or gets rid of symptoms be a problem?

Many addicts have blackouts or memory lapses. They forget things they've said or done while under the influence of alcohol or other drugs. Blackouts can prevent you from recognizing your addiction.

Another factor contributing to denial of addiction is the belief that you "always" have to lose control of alcohol or drug use if you're an addict. The truth is that addiction is characterized by "inconsistent control," not total loss of control in all instances. Every alcoholic doesn't get drunk every single time he or she drinks. Every drug addict doesn't get high or stoned each time he or she uses drugs.

Euphoric recall can fuel the process of denial as well. This refers to remembering only the "positive" aspects of use. You may only remember the feelings of being high, buzzed up, mellow, or euphoric. Or you may only remember "having fun or a good time" even though in reality you made a fool out of yourself and embarrassed or upset other people.

Symptoms of many psychiatric illnesses are lack of insight and poor judgment. As a result of having an illness, you may deny you are sick. For example, people who experience manic or psychotic episodes may not realize that they are sick or are showing behaviors that threaten their safety or the safety of others. People with depression may deny their mood disorder by telling themselves that everyone gets a bad case of the blues once in a while and that they need to pull themselves out of it. And people with certain personality disorders blame all of their behaviors or problems on other people, bad breaks or bad luck, or society.

Recovery Activity

1. List examples of how you denied your psychiatric problem:

   Example: *"I told myself getting busted by the cops happened because of bad luck, not because I was antisocial and breaking the law."*

   _____

   _____

   _____

   _____

2. List examples of how your denial of your addiction showed.

   Example: *"I thought that since pills and booze settled my nerves, how could these be a problem?"*

   _____

   _____

   _____

   _____

3. List other people who denied your addiction and/or psychiatric disorder:

   Example: *"My husband got high with me. He told me all I needed was to cut down and control my drug use better, that I didn't need to stop completely."*

   _____

   _____

   _____

   _____

4. If you continue using alcohol or drugs, how will this affect your psychiatric condition?

_____

_____

_____

_____

5. If you don't get help with your psychiatric disorder, how can this affect your addiction?

_____

_____

_____

_____

SESSION 11
Roadblocks to Recovery

There are many barriers or roadblocks that may interfere with your recovery. You may resist recovery for different reasons. Admitting to a psychiatric problem can be hard. Plus, giving up alcohol and other drugs *and* changing yourself or your lifestyle is not easy. Recovery requires hard work on your part over a long period of time because there are no quick fixes or easy ways to deal with dual disorders.

Recovery roadblocks may relate to your attitudes, beliefs, feelings, and motivation about recovery, your personality traits, your relationships with others, or your lifestyle. Being aware of your roadblocks puts you in a position to do something about them.

1.   I identify with the following recovery roadblocks relating to my attitudes or motivation (✓ all that apply):

   ____   It's hard to admit I have a psychiatric disorder or need professional help.

   ____   I'm worried I can't stay off alcohol or other drugs.

   ____   I don't give a damn about recovery.

   ____   I don't feel very capable or motivated to change.

   ____   My motivation changes from day-to-day.

   ____   I'm very angry at being in treatment.

   ____   I'm only in treatment because of others and I don't want it for myself.

   ____   I don't think staff can help me or understand me.

   ____   I don't trust the staff (doctor, therapist, case manager, etc.).

   ____   I don't stick with AA, NA, CA, dual recovery, or mental health support groups.

   ____   I don't have a sponsor or use the 12-Step program.

   ____   It's hard for me to talk about my "real" problems.

   ____   I don't follow-through with outpatient treatment and miss sessions.

   ____   I don't like taking medications.

2.   I identify with the following recovery roadblocks relating to my personality (✓ all that apply):

   ____   I don't want others telling me what to do.

   ____   I'm stubborn and have to do things my own way.

   ____   It's hard for me to change.

   ____   I'm too impulsive and often act before I think.

____ I'm too perfectionistic.

____ I give up too easily.

____ I depend too much on others to figure out what to do.

____ I use anger or hostility to keep people from getting to know me.

____ I don't open up with others and keep my problems to myself.

3. I identify with the following recovery roadblocks relating to my personal relationships (✓ all that apply):

____ My partner, spouse, or roommate gets high.

____ I live with other family members or friends who get high.

____ Most or all of my friends get high.

____ It's hard for me to relate to people who don't get high.

____ I don't have anyone I can lean on for support.

____ It's hard for me to ask others for help.

____ It's hard for me to trust other people.

____ I don't feel close to anyone.

____ I don't feel loved by anyone.

____ I don't like to listen to authority figures.

4. I identify with the following recovery roadblocks related to my lifestyle (✓ all that apply).

____ My lifestyle centers around getting or using chemicals.

____ I don't have any routine or structure in my life.

____ My living situation is a threat to my recovery.

____ I have little or no direction in my life.

____ I have too much free time on my hands.

____ I live mainly from day-to-day without planning much for the future.

____ I like hanging with a fast crowd, even if I'm not using.

____ My life is a drag and I don't have much to do that is rewarding or fun.

5. My other recovery roadblocks are:

_____

_____

6.   In reviewing the items I checked, here are two personal roadblocks to recovery and ways I can overcome each roadblock:

Roadblock #1 = _____

_____

Ways to overcome this roadblock to my recovery are:

_____

_____

_____

Roadblock # 2 = _____

_____

Ways to overcome this roadblock to my recovery are:

_____

_____

_____

Stan's Roadblock

I have a lot of roadblocks messing with my recovery. I'm tired of going in and out of rehabs, jails, and psychiatric hospitals. Been in too many times to count. Deep down, I'm scared I can't stay clean. But, man, the biggest obstacle to my recovery is me. I copped a bad attitude about treatment and other people telling me what to do to stop getting high and messing up my life. In treatment, I talk like I know what's going down. But ain't nothing gonna get better unless I do what they say in NA—quit talking the talk and get on with walking the walk. So here's what I'm gonna do: get a sponsor and use him, go to meetings every day, and keep my mouth shut and listen to find out what recovery's all about. I'm going to keep all of my counseling sessions and stop BS-ing about why I shouldn't go. It ain't that hard—just be responsible and don't do things my way. My way just don't work, so it's time to try another way.

SESSION 12
Recovery from Dual Disorders

Recovery from dual disorders involves addressing your psychiatric illness, your addiction, and the problems contributing to or resulting from your disorders. Recovery is a *long-term process* that requires effort on your part and a willingness to get actively involved in improving yourself. It involves:

- Getting sober or clean from alcohol or drugs
- Stabilizing from acute psychiatric symptoms
- Learning information about your illnesses, treatment of them, and what all is involved in recovery
- Motivating yourself to change because you want to get well
- Developing realistic attitudes about recovery and change
- Developing skills to stay sober from alcohol or drugs
- Developing skills to cope with your psychiatric problems
- Actively working a recovery program that focuses on your dual disorders and making positive changes in yourself and your lifestyle
- Developing a relapse prevention plan

Recovery = Abstinence + Specific Treatment + Change

Recovery Involves: • information • attitudes • motivation • skills • a program

---

Phases of Recovery

There are different phases of recovery. Each phase has some key issues that are fairly common to people recovering from dual disorders. However, not every person progresses through these phases in the same way or at the same rate, so keep this in mind as you read about these phases of recovery. Factors determining your progression include the severity of your disorders and your personality, coping style, support network, and motivation to work a recovery program.

Phase 1 — Transition and Engagement

This phase of recovery involves becoming engaged in treatment, either voluntarily or as a result of an involuntary commitment. This involves some recognition that you haven't been able to control your use of alcohol or other drugs, or that your psychiatric disorder requires treatment. However, in cases of involuntary commitment involving severe psychiatric decompensation, recognition may not occur until there is some stability of your acute psychiatric symptoms.

Your alcohol or drug use may have played a major role in a new episode of psychiatric illness following a period of remission. Or your chemical use may have led to a worsening of existing psychiatric symptoms such as depression, mania, psychosis, suicidality, anxiety, panic, out-of-control or threatening behaviors toward others, or an inability to function very well and take care of your basic needs. In some cases your alcohol or drug use may have "masked" your psychiatric symptoms, prolonging your entry into treatment.

During this transition and engagement phase, you begin to recognize that an untreated psychiatric disorder interferes with your ability to remain sober from alcohol or other drugs or negatively affects your motivation and desire to recover from addiction. This phase involves engaging in professional treatment in a psychiatric hospital or outpatient setting, or an addiction rehabilitation setting, depending on the nature and severity of your symptoms. If you enter treatment through a psychiatric system, you may eventually be referred to an addiction rehabilitation program if it is thought that this is essential for you to initiate your recovery from addiction.

In this phase you begin to come to grips with your mixed feelings about recovery, accepting the reality that part of you wants to stop using chemicals and get well and part of you doesn't want to stop using chemicals or make any changes. The same holds true for your psychiatric illness—you begin to accept that part of you needs help and part of you doesn't think you need any help, that you can get well on your own.

If possible, your family should get involved in your treatment. They can provide helpful information to professionals who care for you, emotional support to you, and they can gain much from treatment for themselves. The earlier they get involved in the assessment and treatment processes, the better it usually is for everyone involved.

You also begin to accept the need for a recovery program that involves a combination of professional treatment and self-help programs such as AA, NA, CA, DRA, or other mental health support groups. You learn that you need help and support from others in order to recover from your dual disorders. Your motivation to change initially may be "external" during this recovery phase as you get involved in recovery mainly because of the problems your addiction and mental health disorder have caused, or because you have been "forced" or "pressured" to accept help by your family, employer, the court system, a health care or social service professional, or some other important person in your life.

This transition and engagement phase may take several weeks or longer, although for some it takes months or years to become truly engaged in dual diagnosis recovery and motivated to change. Some enter treatment only to drop out early. If you make a commitment to stay in recovery, even if you feel your motivation is questionable, you put yourself in a good position to benefit from treatment. Keep in mind that many people need time to develop their motivation to recover, and that staying in treatment "buys you time" to develop this motivation and see the many potential benefits of treatment.

Phase 2 — Stabilization

This phase involves stabilizing from your acute psychiatric symptoms. In this phase you may receive medications to help stabilize your psychiatric symptoms. Depending on the nature of your symptoms and your past response to medications, it may take several weeks or even longer for medications to work effectively in reducing or eliminating your symptoms. This requires patience on your part and a willingness to stick with treatment even if you feel frustrated. In some cases, stabilizing from an episode of psychiatric illness is a relatively smooth process. In other cases, it is much more complex and takes longer.

The stabilization phase also involves getting alcohol and drugs out of your system and adjusting to being chemically free. For some people detoxification in an inpatient or outpatient setting is needed to break the cycle of addictive chemical use. **Acute symptoms** of withdrawal from alcohol or other drugs usually last only a few days to a week or so. The specific withdrawal symptoms you may experience depend on the amount and types of chemicals you have been using. **Protracted (or post acute withdrawal) symptoms**, on the other hand, may last for weeks or months. If your body was used to heavy use of alcohol or other drugs for years, you can't expect it to adjust to being chemically free in just a few short days.

Essential components of this stabilization process are acquiring information about your illnesses and the role of professional therapy, medications, and self-help programs in ongoing recovery. The more you learn, the more empowered you will feel. And the more aware you will become of the course of recovery as it relates to the specific illnesses that you have as well as what you need to do to help yourself. In this phase you should learn about your specific diagnoses, causes of psychiatric and addictive illnesses, effects of dual disorders, and steps you can take to help yourself cope with your disorders.

In this phase of recovery, you begin to learn ways to cope with your addictive thinking, cravings to use alcohol or drugs and symptoms of your psychiatric illness. In addition to involvement in professional treatment, you get involved in self-help programs such as AA, NA, CA for your addiction; Double Trouble, MISA, SAMI, CAMI or Dual Recovery Anonymous programs for your dual disorders; or special mental support groups based on the nature of your specific psychiatric illness (for example, anxiety disorder support groups, manic-depression support groups, etc.).

As you progress through this phase of recovery, you become less preoccupied with alcohol and other drugs. You learn ways to counteract euphoric recall and other positive thoughts about using chemicals so that you reduce your risk of relapsing. You also learn that recovery is possible and, despite whatever psychiatric illness you have, there are effective treatments. Your motivation gets stronger in this phase as you learn that there are many steps you can take to help your recovery. Very importantly, you become more comfortable accepting help and support from others such as professionals, sponsors and members of support programs, and your family.

A major aspect of this phase is accepting the need for long-term involvement in professional treatment and self-help recovery. You work closely with your treatment team in developing a list of problems that you need to work on, prioritizing these problems, and developing problem-solving strategies to begin addressing select problems from your list. You accept the need for total abstinence from alcohol, street drugs, and nonprescribed drugs.

Your family's involvement should continue in this phase as well. The degree and nature of their involvement depends on your needs, their needs, and the recommendations of the professionals providing treatment to you. Excluding your family from ongoing involvement in recovery can lead to serious problems later.

This phase of recovery may take up to several months. The ease in which you move through this stage depends on the severity of your psychiatric illness and your addiction, as well as the type of treatment that you are receiving. Again, the importance of addressing both your addiction and your psychiatric illness must be stressed because it will be extremely hard to stabilize if both disorders aren't addressed in your recovery.

Phase 3 — Early Recovery

This phase of recovery involves continued work at recovery from both of your disorders. You work at staying sober by learning some practical ways of coping with cravings and desires to use chemicals. And you learn to avoid people, places, and things that represent a relapse risk for you. Because you cannot avoid all risk factors, you slowly begin to learn nonchemical ways of coping with pressures from others to use alcohol or other drugs, and coping with situations that in the past led you to using chemicals. You become more used to sobriety and coping with the many physical, emotional, and social adjustments it brings. During this phase you begin to make internal changes by learning how to combat your addictive thinking. You also begin incorporating new sobriety-based values that help you strengthen your commitment to abstinence. Your "sober" side takes a stronger role than your "addicted" side and you more openly embrace the need for a recovery program that accepts total abstinence as the best goal for you. You still want to use at times but you know this is part of addictive disease and that you can cope with this part if you use the tools of the program that you have been learning.

During early recovery you begin to learn ways of coping with your psychiatric disorder and the problems it may have caused in your life. You learn that while medication can help improve some of the symptoms of your illness, you have to work hard at making changes in yourself and your lifestyle in order to promote a better recovery. You learn to challenge and change negative thinking that previously contributed to anxiety, depression, or unhappiness. You become more realistic about recovery and the need for active involvement in a program of change. During this phase you also learn to change some of your behaviors, especially ones that caused you difficulties in the past. You increase your awareness of the role of your behaviors, thinking, and personality in your psychiatric disorder.

Early recovery also involves building structure and regularity into your day-to-day life so that you keep busy, stay focused on recovery issues, get involved in leisure activities that are enjoyable, and don't have a lot of free time on your hands. Structure helps you stay focused on your goals and can serve as a protective factor against relapse to your psychiatric illness or your addiction.

In family sessions you focus on understanding the impact of your disorders and behaviors on your family. You learn how they can support your recovery and how you can support them. You and your family learn to communicate more openly about recovery. This helps set the stage for making amends later on.

Involvement in therapy and support programs help you with these issues. Working the 12 Steps becomes an important aspect of your change plan. So does working with a sponsor who can guide you in using the "tools" of recovery.

As you progress through this stage, you feel less guilty and shameful because you learn that you are not a "bad person" but that your disorders contributed to behaviors that were problematic for you and others. You accept responsibility for coping with your disorders by staying involved in professional treatment and self-help programs. It becomes clear that you need continued help and support from others since recovery has so many challenges.

Early recovery roughly involves three to six months after the stabilization phase. Similar to previous phases, some work through this phase more easily than others. If you relapse to alcohol or drug use, or experience a worsening of your psychiatric symptoms during this phase, you will need to restabilize before you can address the issues discussed above.

Phase 4 — Middle Recovery

This phase involves building on the work from the previous early recovery phase. In therapy, you share more about your inner thoughts and feelings and reach a greater level of self-awareness. You work on improving your interpersonal relationships. This requires learning to communicate more openly with others and nurturing your relationships with family, friends, or other significant people in your life. You become more caring and loving toward others. You not only *get* support and help from others, but you also *give* to others, too. This helps you develop more balanced relationships.

In middle recovery you spend more time and effort repairing the damage to your relationships and self-esteem caused by your dual disorders. Steps 8 and 9 of AA, NA, CA, or DRA are addressed with your sponsor and/or therapist. These steps help you identify others hurt by your behaviors, become willing to make amends, and figure out ways to make amends in cases where doing so will not bring harm to other people. Your relationships become more meaningful and satisfying as a result. In relationships where damage cannot be repaired and the relationships cannot be salvaged, you learn to accept this reality rather than judge yourself harshly.

Spirituality issues in recovery become more important during this phase. You further develop your own unique sense of spirituality and use this to help your recovery and growth as a person. This process may or may not also involve active participation in some formal type of religion. As you progress through this phase of recovery, you focus more on becoming a better person and being satisfied with yourself. Steps 10 and 11, in particular, help in this process.

You continue improving how you cope with negative or upsetting thoughts and feelings during middle recovery. You learn to change anxious, depressed, or other negative thinking patterns. You realize that by changing your thinking, you can change your feelings as well as how you act. Your coping strategies strengthen as you practice new ways of thinking, feeling, and behaving. As you make changes in different areas of yourself and your life, your self-esteem rises. You feel less demoralized and victimized by your disorders. Instead, you see the need to continue responsibly making changes in yourself. You stop blaming society, bad breaks, bad genes, or others for your problems.

Because addictive and psychiatric disorders are often chronic, relapsing illnesses, you learn to identify and manage warning signs of relapse during this recovery phase. You learn that going back to using alcohol and drugs doesn't usually "come out of the blue" but represents a movement away from recovery toward relapse over a period of time. Similarly, you learn that new episodes of psychiatric illness or significant worsening of persistent and chronic psychiatric symptoms often occur gradually over time. Knowing your potential relapse warning signs allows you to develop recovery strategies that reduce the likelihood of relapse to either or both of your disorders. Your relapse prevention plan becomes an important part of recovery. By monitoring your recovery on a daily basis, you put yourself in a position to spot relapse warning signs early. This, in turn, allows you to take action before things get out of hand.

If your psychiatric illness was a first episode and you are fairly free of symptoms as a result of treatment, you may be withdrawn from medications. Usually this is not done until you have been doing well for four months or longer. If you have a recurrent psychiatric disorder or a chronic, persistent form of illness such as schizophrenia or bipolar disease, you most likely will remain on medications even if you are doing well. The purpose of medications in such a case is to *prevent* the possibility of a recurrence of psychiatric illness. The idea is similar to taking medications for high blood pressure or other medical illnesses: taking medicine maintains treatment gains and helps prevent future symptoms. It still is possible for symptoms to break through even if you continue to take medications. However, this happens less often than in cases where medications are stopped prematurely. Middle recovery usually involves the six- to twelve-month period following early recovery. Again, as in other phases, some people move through this phase more easily than others.

Phase 5 — Late Recovery

This phase of recovery involves continued work started in the previous phases. Usually, you get into personal recovery issues in greater depth during this phase as you have established a solid foundation for your recovery. You focus more on changing your "character defects" and dealing with other problems caused by your personality style. You build on your strengths and work on your weaknesses.

Late recovery involves working at finding greater meaning in life and developing more positive values. The spiritual and interpersonal aspects of recovery help you in this quest. One of the many beautiful aspects of recovery is that it provides you a chance to become a better, more fulfilled person. But this only comes with patience, discipline, and hard work.

If you are in therapy, focus may shift away from practical daily life issues and more toward greater self-exploration so that you better understand yourself—your defenses, personality style, patterns of behavior, values, and strengths. You gain greater clarity on how your past influences you at the present time. Greater self-understanding helps to pave the way for you to make personal changes and improve yourself.

As you progress through this phase, you become more able and willing to focus on healing from past emotional wounds related to growing up in a family in which a serious addiction or mental health problem existed, or related to other traumatic experiences such as incest or other forms of abuse. You learn to face your pain head-on rather than use it as a reason to drink alcohol or use drugs, or as a reason not to change your life. Gradually you let go of your anger, disappointment, and sadness. And you begin to learn to forgive others you feel harmed you in the past. If you are unable or unwilling to forgive, you learn to live with your pain and anger in ways that aren't self-destructive.

In some instances this healing takes place by working the 12-Step program of AA, NA, CA, or DRA. In other cases it involves deeper exploration in therapy sessions. Therapy helps you slowly work through your pain and put it in a different perspective so that it doesn't continue to cause you so much emotional pain. To aid your healing journey, you may also participate in other types of self-help support groups such as Adult Children of Alcoholics, Incest Survivors Anonymous, or codependency groups.

Late recovery also gives you the opportunity to work at "balancing" the various areas of your life—recovery, work, love, relationships, fun, and spirituality. This phase roughly involves a year to two after the middle recovery period.

Phase 6 — Maintenance

This final phase is best seen as an *ongoing* phase. It involves continued work on your "self" through ongoing work at a recovery program. You shift toward more self-reliance during this phase and rely less on others for help and support. You still need and depend on others, but more and more you rely on your own inner resources to cope with your thoughts, feelings, and problems in life.

Part of your continued growth and development may come from "giving away" what you learned in recovery by sponsoring others and working Step 12. You are able to use your experience, hope, and strength to help others in recovery.

Because you are well-grounded in recovery by this time, you are better able to deal with the problems life brings you in your day-to-day life. You face these head-on, whatever they are. Coping with problems and changes in your life doesn't overwhelm you like it did in the early phases of recovery.

You learn to cope with setbacks and mistakes that you make in your life and recovery. You use your mistakes to learn something new about yourself or life rather than as a reason to put yourself down. You become more accepting of your limitations, weaknesses, and flaws. You modify your goals in life if you discover you cannot reach them or that they were too high in the first place.

During the maintenance phase, if you have a recurrent or persistent form of psychiatric illness, you continue taking medications. By this phase you probably have decreased the frequency you see a therapist or psychiatrist as you are busy "living the program" of recovery.

As the name of this phase implies, it is ongoing. You "maintain" gains made previously while continuing to grow as a person. If you have a setback and relapse to your addiction or psychiatric illness, you won't necessarily have to go through all of these phases again. This all depends on the nature of your relapse, how long it lasts, and the damage it does to you and your relationships. And, as I said before, these phases are simply "rough guides" to help you understand the recovery process. Try to avoid comparing yourself to others because everyone works differently in recovery. Measure your progress in relation to previous periods of illness. Even if you are still having problems, it is possible that you still are making progress and moving in the right direction. Remember, progress sometimes comes in small steps.

You will do better in recovery if you actively work your treatment plan and follow through with it. You increase the chances of getting well and making positive changes by attending your treatment sessions with your doctor, therapist, and/or group, taking your medications, attending support group meetings, getting and using a sponsor, and asking your family to get involved.

Areas of Recovery

In the preceding sections I discussed some examples of change that are associated with various phases of recovery. Another way to look at your recovery plan is to think about the different areas of your life and to identify specific changes that you want to make. Your recovery plan may involve any of the following areas:

- **Physical** — ensuring that you get enough sleep and rest, eating nutritious meals and eating regularly, exercising to keep in shape and release built-up tension, learning how to relax and manage stress, and dealing with cravings or strong desires to use alcohol or drugs.

- **Emotional** — working through your denial and accepting both of your disorders and the need to change; developing skills to cope with your feelings, thoughts, and problems; working through emotional wounds from the past; improving your self-esteem; and coping with persistent symptoms of your illness.

- **Family and interpersonal** — evaluating the impact of your disorders and behaviors on your family and other people, making amends when appropriate, building a recovery support system and healthy relationships, encouraging your family to get involved in treatment sessions with you and/or support groups for families (Alanon, Naranon, Families of the Mentally Ill, etc.), improving your communication skills, and improving the quality of your relationships.

- **Social and leisure** — spending time involved in social and leisure activities that bring you enjoyment and satisfaction; making sure that you don't isolate yourself from other people; avoiding people, places, and things associated with getting drunk or high; learning how to say no when other people offer you alcohol or drugs; and learning how to have fun without needing alcohol or drugs.

- **Lifestyle** — building structure and routine into your daily life so you keep busy and are engaged in constructive work, leisure, social, or recovery activities; learning how to manage money; setting goals that you want to work toward achieving; and dealing with any legal, financial, job, school, or other problems.

- **Spiritual** — developing your spiritual or religious beliefs, becoming active in your religion, relying on God or your Higher Power for inner strength, and praying or reading the Bible or other spiritual materials.

- **Daily inventory** — monitoring your progress on a daily basis in order to keep track of your symptoms and problems to determine if you are getting better or sliding backward. A daily inventory helps you catch relapse warning signs and problems early so you can face them head-on rather than wait until things build up too much.

Answer the following questions related to the recovery process from dual disorders:

1.   Which phase of recovery do you think you are in?   Explain your answer.

_____

_____

_____

_____

_____

2.   Of the areas of recovery discussed, list two that are most important to you at this time.   Then, for each one, list steps you can take to work on these two recovery issues.

Recovery Issue #1 = _____

_____

Steps to Take:

_____

_____

_____

_____

_____

Recovery Issue #2 = _____

_____

Steps to Take:

_____

_____

_____

_____

_____

SESSION 13
Coping with Cravings for Alcohol or Drugs

Cravings for alcohol or other drugs are common when you first stop using. One craving may be so strong and intense that you feel like you'll go crazy if you don't get drugs. Another craving may be no big deal.

Your cravings may be overt, which means you know you are craving alcohol or drugs. Or your cravings may be covert or "hidden," which means you don't know you want alcohol or drugs. For example, some people become very irritable, upset, and edgy when they first enter a hospital or rehabilitation program. They become critical of staff, other patients, and recovery. Some even check themselves out against medical advice. In many cases what lies beneath the surface and is a major reason for this irritability or edginess is a hidden craving for alcohol or drugs.

Cravings are triggered by many different **internal factors** such as feeling anxious, angry, or edgy. **External factors** that trigger cravings include people, places, events, things or objects, rituals, or experiences that remind you of using or being high. Sometimes you don't need anything to trigger it; your addiction itself can cause cravings.

It helps to know the common triggers that cause alcohol or drug cravings. It also helps to figure out your own craving triggers. Once you know your triggers and how your cravings show, you can then develop coping strategies to help you cope with a craving so that you don't use chemicals. The following exercise shows you one way to understand your alcohol and drug cravings.

Answer the following to help understand your craving triggers and signs:

1. My **internal craving triggers** are:

    *   *Feelings*

        _____

        _____

    *   *Thoughts*

        _____

        _____

    *   *Physical sensations or symptoms*

        _____

        _____

2. Factors in my environment (**external triggers**) that cause cravings to get high are:

- *People (other users, spouse or partner, the pusher/dealer, etc.).*

_____

_____

- *Places (bars or clubs, certain peoples' homes, crack houses, bathroom at work, car, street corners, etc.).*

_____

_____

- *Events or experiences associated with using (parties, sporting events, payday, check day, etc.).*

_____

_____

- *Things or objects associated with using or preparing chemicals (seeing or smelling alcohol or other drugs; ads for beer, wine or liquor; needles, coke spoons, papers, pipes, and bongs; mirrors, credit cards, vials, scales, music, money, etc.).*

_____

_____

- *Other situations (getting a flu shot, visiting a doctor, etc.).*

_____

_____

3. Do you still have drugs or paraphernalia (pipes, needles, etc.) in your home?

____ Yes ____ No. If yes, why and what are you going to do with them?

_____

_____

4. Do you keep alcohol in your home?

____ Yes ____ No. If yes, why and what are you going to do with it?

_____

_____

5. Think of three recent times you experienced cravings for alcohol or other drugs. Rate each of these on a scale of 1 to 10 by placing a ✓ for each craving.

	1 Not Intense	3 Somewhat Intense	5 Pretty Intense	7 Very Intense	10 Extremely Intense
Craving 1					
Craving 2					
Craving 3					

6. Five to ten positive ways to help me resist the desire to use when I crave alcohol or drugs are:

_____

_____

_____

_____

_____

_____

_____

_____

_____

_____

7. If I am able to cope successfully with cravings I will feel:

_____

_____

_____

8. If I give in to my cravings I will feel:

_____

_____

_____

Carol's Triggers and Plan

I have a lot of triggers to get high. When I feel real pissed or upset, I get strong desires to use drugs. Plus, when I'm around JJ, Marsha, Petey, Maria, and some other people I partied with, I think about using. It's almost automatic.

What am I going to do? When I'm mad or upset, I'll talk things over with my sponsor or NA friends either on the phone or in person. I'll argue with that little voice in my head that tells me to go ahead and use drugs. I'll tell it to go to hell, that I ain't going to use under no circumstances. I got rid of all the booze and drugs in my house. I'm not going to hang with people I partied with and I got the word out I'm not using no more. I'm only hanging out with people who don't get high because it's too dangerous to be with addicts who aren't in recovery. At the start of each day, I'm going to remind myself why I should stay clean today.

Craving Busters

- *Recognize and label your craving.*

The previous section provided information that should help you know the signs of your cravings as well as the triggers. Use whatever label is comfortable for you: craving, desire, urge, or drug or alcohol hunger.

- *Talk about your craving.*

Talk with your sponsor, an AA, NA, or CA friend, counselor, close friend, or family member. This may provide relief, and you may hear from others how they coped with cravings. Sometimes talking may increase your craving. If this happens to you, use other coping strategies.

- *Go to a self-help meeting (AA, NA, CA, etc).*

This can provide you with an opportunity to discuss your craving with others and hear how they have coped with theirs.

- *Use self-talk.*

Tell yourself you won't use or that you'll put off using for a few hours or days. By that time your craving will have passed. Think positive and tell yourself you'll get through your craving. Remind yourself of the benefits of not using and problems if you use again. Imagine that you can talk to your craving and tell it to "go to hell," that you won't let it defeat you. Remind yourself that the more struggles with cravings you win, the stronger you will feel.

- *Accept that in time it will pass.*

  Sometimes all you need to do is accept the fact that cravings will come and go. You don't have to use just because you have a craving. Remember, *it will pass.*

- *Do something active — now!*

  This can help redirect your energies and divert your attention. Make a list of activities you can keep busy with if your craving gets strong. Hobbies, sports, or other physical activities can help you cope with your cravings.

- *Write in a journal.*

  Put your thoughts and feelings into words and write them in a journal. You can describe your cravings and the situations in which they occur. You can also keep track of the outcome of your craving and positive coping strategies you used. Keeping a regular journal may even help you figure out if there are patterns to your cravings.

- *Get rid of booze, drugs, and paraphernalia.*

  Don't keep alcohol and drugs in your home. Get rid of drug paraphernalia such as papers, pipes, needles, mirrors, etc.

- *Keep a craving coping card in your wallet or purse.*

  Write down a list of positive coping strategies and carry this on a 3" X 5" index card in your wallet or purse. Review this to remind yourself of positive strategies to deal with cravings.

- *Be aware of high-risk people, places, and situations.*

  There may be people, places, or situations you must avoid to not put yourself at risk to use, especially during times when you feel a strong craving. Because you can't avoid all high-risk people or situations, you need to be prepared ahead of time so that you can cope with cravings or desires to use if they pop up.

- *Pray.*

  Ask God or your Higher Power for help and strength to get through your craving.

- *Read recovery literature.*

  Read passages from the AA "Big Book," the NA "Basic Text," *Learning to Live Again: A Guide for Recovery from Chemical Dependency* (Miller, Gorski, and Miller), or other books and guides on recovery. Reading may provide you with coping strategies, inspire you to continue your recovery journey, or calm yourself down. See the list at the end of this workbook in the Appendix for some suggested readings.

SECTION IV

Building Emotional Strength

SESSION 14
Coping with Anger

Anger problems are common among people with dual disorders. Much friction can be caused in a relationship if you ignore your anger or act on it in ways that hurt others physically or emotionally. Anger problems can interfere with your recovery if you don't cope with these feelings in positive ways.

Anger can also empower you if you deal with it in a positive way. It can motivate you to set or reach goals or work hard to accomplish things in your life.

It is not your feelings of anger that cause problems but how you think about and express it that determines how anger affects your life. Some people try to ignore their anger and let it build up. They stew on the inside and become upset or depressed. They express anger indirectly by dragging their feet, forgetting important dates of people they feel anger toward, criticizing others behind their backs, or avoiding people they are mad at.

Other people let their anger out much too quickly and impulsively. They lash out at others and yell, cuss, scream, or act in other hostile ways. Some get into fights or destroy objects or property.

The questions that follow will help you assess your anger and how you express it:

1. On a scale of 1 to 10, how much of a problem is your anger or how you cope with it or express it (✓ your rating).

1	*3*	*5*	*7*	*10*
No	*Moderate*	*Significant*	*Serious*	*Severe*
Problem	*Problem*	*Problem*	*Problem*	*Problem*

    _____   _____   _____   _____   _____

2. My anger usually shows in the following ways (for example, I get sad, frustrated, pace, and feel nervous, etc.).

    _____

    _____

    _____

    _____

3. I usually deal with anger by: (for example, holding it inside, letting it out immediately, talking it out, lashing out at others, fighting, etc.).

_____

_____

_____

_____

4. I learned the following from my parents about anger or how to express it:

_____

_____

_____

_____

5. My anger affects my physical or mental health in the following ways:

_____

_____

_____

_____

6. My anger affects my relationships in the following ways:

_____

_____

_____

_____

7. My anger affects my use of alcohol or other drugs by:

_____

_____

_____

8. I am still very angry at the following people:

_____

_____

_____

9. I can use my anger in a positive way by:

_____

_____

_____

Setting a Goal

My *Goal* in relation to how I cope with my anger is:

_____

_____

***Steps* I will take to reach this goal are:**

_____

_____

***Potential benefits* of reaching my goal are:**

_____

_____

Anger Busters

- *Recognize your angry feelings.*

  Pay attention to body cues, thoughts, and behaviors telling you that you are angry. Use your anger cues to admit that you are angry. Don't deny, hide, minimize, or ignore your anger.

- *Figure out why you are angry.*

  When you feel angry, figure out of where it is coming from. Does it relate to something another person did or said to you? Does it relate to an event, experience, or situation? Or is your anger caused by the way you think about things?

- *Decide if you really should feel angry.*

  Are you an angry person who seems to get mad too often or for no good reason? When angry, ask yourself if the facts of the situation warrant an angry reaction on your part. Or ask yourself if your anger is the result of a character defect (for example, you get mad frequently for little things).

- *Identify the effects of your anger and your methods of coping with anger.*

  How does your anger and your methods of coping with it affect your physical, mental, or spiritual health? How are your relationships with family members, friends, or others affected?

- *Use different strategies to deal with anger.*

  These include *cognitive* (your beliefs about anger and the internal messages you give yourself), *behavioral* (how you act), and *verbal* (what you say to other people) strategies. Having a variety of strategies puts you in a good position to cope with anger in a wide range of situations.

- *COGNITIVE STRATEGIES for anger management include:*

  • Evaluating your beliefs about anger and changing those beliefs that cause you problems. For example, if you believe you should "let it out" every time you get angry, you may find this isn't always the best policy and that this belief should be modified. Or if you believe you should never get mad, you might have to change this belief and give yourself permission to feel anger.

  • Catching yourself when you are angry and changing your angry thoughts.

• Determining if your anger is really justified given the situation. This requires not jumping to conclusions and getting all the facts of the situation first.

• Using positive self-talk or slogans (for example, "This too will pass," "Keep your cool and stay in control").

• Using fantasy—imagine yourself coping in a positive way.

• Evaluating the risks and benefits of expressing your anger or holding it inside.

• Reminding yourself of negative effects of ignoring anger and holding it inside.

• Reminding yourself of negative effects of expressing anger toward others in hurtful ways.

• Identifying the benefits of handling anger in a positive way.

• Taking a few minutes at the end of the day to see if you are harboring any anger from the events of the day.

• *VERBAL STRATEGIES for anger management include:*

  • Sharing your feelings with the one you are angry with.

  • Discussing the situation or problem that contributed to your anger directly with the one you are angry with.

  • Sharing your angry feelings with a friend, family member, therapist, or sponsor (AA, NA, or CA). Many find it helpful to discuss anger at support group meetings.

  • Discussing the situation or problem that contributed to your anger with a neutral person to get their opinion on the situation.

  • Apologizing or making amends to others who were hurt as a result of how you expressed your anger.

- *BEHAVIOR STRATEGIES for anger management include:*

  • Directing angry energy toward physical activity such as walking, exercise, or sports.

  • Directing feelings of anger toward some type of work.

  • Expressing your anger with creative media such as painting, drawing, and other forms of arts and crafts.

  • Writing about your feelings in a journal or anger log.

  • Practicing verbal strategies mentioned in the previous section so you feel better prepared to express your feelings to others.

  • Using reminder cards that provide you with specific coping strategies you can use to deal with anger.

  • Leaving situations in which your anger is so intense you worry about losing control and doing something irrational or violent.

Seek professional help if you experience serious problems as a result of anger and how you cope with it, or if you are unable to gain better control of it on your own. Professional help is especially important for those who act out angry impulses by hitting or hurting others or breaking objects. Professional treatment also can help those who turn anger against themselves and exhibit self-destructive tendencies such as those who cut, burn, or hurt themselves.

SESSION 15
Coping with Anxiety and Worry

Most people feel anxious and worry at times. However, some people experience excessive anxiety and worry so much that it causes a lot of distress in their lives. Anxiety symptoms are common among people with addiction, serious depression, or other psychiatric disorders. Many use alcohol or drugs to decrease their anxiety only to find in the long run such use leads to chemical dependency, or they avoid situations that cause their anxious feelings. Anxiety is quite common when a person first stops drinking alcohol or using drugs. It is a common withdrawal symptom and has both a physical and psychological basis.

Anxiety refers to the *physical* side and worry refers to the *mental* side. When you have one, you usually have the other. Anxiety shows in physical symptoms such as: shortness of breath, rapid heart beat, tightness or discomfort in the chest, feeling lightheaded or weak, feeling uptight or on edge, or tingling and numbness.

Anticipatory anxiety refers to feeling anxious when you think ahead of time what "may happen" at some event or situation in the future. Some people avoid situations because of this. Some situations they may avoid include: shopping in a large or crowded store; standing in checkout lines in stores; writing in public; going to the doctor or dentist; attending church, movies, sporting events, or music concerts; driving through tunnels or over bridges; riding elevators or escalators; or traveling by plane, bus, or train. Some people become so anxious and fearful of leaving home that they seldom or never leave home. When they do leave home, they often need another person to go along with them.

Worry refers to thinking about things over and over in your head in relation to a *real* problem or a *potential* problem (something that you think might happen). People who worry a lot often feel inadequate in being able to cope with the problems or situations they worry about.

The questions that follow will help you assess your level of anxiety and worry:

1. On a scale of 1 to 10, how much of a problem is your anxiety, or how you cope with it (✓ your rating).

1	*3*	*5*	*7*	*10*
No Problem	*Moderate Problem*	*Significant Problem*	*Serious Problem*	*Severe Problem*
_____	_____	_____	_____	_____

78

2. On a scale of 1 to 10, how much of a problem is your worry, or how you cope with it (✓ your rating).

1	3	5	7	10
No	*Moderate*	*Significant*	*Serious*	*Severe*
Problem	*Problem*	*Problem*	*Problem*	*Problem*
_____	_____	_____	_____	_____

If your ratings were three or higher for either of these, you should consider seeking professional help. If your ratings were five or higher, you should definitely seek professional help with a mental health specialist who also understands addiction.

3. My anxiety shows in the following ways:

_____

_____

_____

_____

_____

4. The reasons I get anxious are:

_____

_____

_____

_____

_____

5. My feelings of anxiety and worry have affected my life in the following ways:

_____

_____

_____

_____

6. My anxiety and worry has affected my relationships in the following ways:

_____

_____

_____

_____

7. I worry a lot about these situations or events:

_____

_____

_____

_____

8. The connection between my use of alcohol or other drugs and my anxiety or worry is:

_____

_____

_____

_____

Setting a Goal

My *Goal* **in relation to my anxiety or worry is:**

_____

_____

Steps **I will take to reach this goal are:**

_____

_____

_____

Potential benefits **of reaching my goal are:**

_____

_____

_____

Anxiety and Worry: Coping Strategies

- **Identify and label anxiety and worry.**

   Know the signs and symptoms of excessive anxiety or worry. This will help you catch yourself when you feel anxious or are worrying too much. Read resources such as *Learning to Live Again* and others listed in the Appendix

- **Find out what is causing your anxiety and worry.**

   Identify the specific problems, situations, or things that cause you to feel anxious and worried. If these are *real* problems, look at ways to solve them. If these are *potential* problems ask yourself if these problems will really occur. Work on changing how you think about potential problems.

- **Get a physical examination.**

   This will help determine if medical problems are contributing to your anxiety.

- **Evaluate your diet.**

  Take a close look at what you are eating or taking into your body. Try to figure out if your use of caffeine, sugar, or other foods is contributing to anxiety and making you feel on edge.

- **Evaluate your lifestyle.**

  Make sure you are getting enough rest, relaxation, and exercise. Exercise can help release some of your anxious feelings. It may serve the additional benefit of helping to prevent anxious feelings from building up.

- **Meditate.**

  This can help you feel calmer and gain better control over your anxiety.

- **Learn relaxation techniques.**

  There are many books and tapes available to help you teach yourself relaxation, or you can learn relaxation techniques from a professional therapist.

- **Practice proper breathing techniques.**

  Stop shallow or rapid breathing or holding your breath. Learn proper ways of breathing and practice these each day until they become automatic. You can practice breathing techniques anywhere—at work, home, in the car, before a speech, or before going into a situation about which you feel anxious.

- **Change your beliefs or thoughts.**

  Practice changing your "anxious" and "worrisome" thoughts or beliefs. When working on a *real* problem causing your anxiety or worry, view the problem for what it is. Don't see it as a barrier that you can't overcome. When feeling real anxious or worried about a *potential* problem, ask yourself what evidence you have that the problem will ever occur or the outcome will be what you fear it will be. Try to identify all possible outcomes, not just the negative ones that you worry will happen. Make positive self-statements such as "I can do it," "My anxiety won't get the best of me," "I'm in control of my worry," "It's OK to make mistakes," or "No one has to be perfect."

- **Share your anxious feelings and thoughts with others.**

  Discussing your feelings and worries with a friend, family member, sponsor, or counselor may help you feel better and gain relief. This can also help you learn what others do to handle their anxiety and worry and identify new ways to cope. However, keep in mind that you can overwhelm others if you constantly share your worries. If you share your feelings and don't make attempts at getting better, you might turn others off. People usually don't mind hearing their friend's or loved one's feelings unless the same old story is told over and over.

- **Set aside "worry time" each day.**

Try to avoid worrying throughout the day and save your worries for a time of the day you call your "worry time." Pick a place and regular time and then allow yourself to let your worries out. Don't go on endlessly; limit yourself to no more than one-half hour a day for this worry time.

- **Keep a written anxiety-and-worry journal.**

Writing your thoughts and feelings in a journal will help you release and better understand your thoughts and feelings. This can help you identify patterns to your anxiety and worry, coping strategies that don't work, and coping strategies that work in reducing anxiety and worry. This can also help you track your progress over time.

- **Face the situations causing you to feel anxious and worried.**

Reality is often not as bad as what you think it will be. When you directly face the situations you find difficult, your confidence level should increase. Start with the least threatening anxiety or worry-provoking situations and gradually build up toward facing the more difficult ones. Engaging in situations you feel anxious and worry about should reduce your anxiety and worry.

- **If your anxiety level continues to cause you significant distress, seek a consultation with a mental health professional.**

A consultation with a mental health professional (psychiatrist, psychologist, social worker, counselor, etc.) will help you determine if your anxiety is a symptom of a psychiatric illness. Many types of treatment are available to help individuals with anxiety disorders. These include different types of psychotherapy as well as medication. Be careful about types of medication used as it is easy to become dependent on medications such as tranquilizers. Let your doctor know that you are recovering from a chemical dependency so that the proper medications are used should your symptoms be serious enough to require the use of medicine.

SESSION 16
Coping with Boredom

Many people say that feelings of boredom give them an excuse to drink alcohol or use other drugs. If your lifestyle was wrapped up in alcohol or drugs, or in the "fast life," being clean or sober may feel very boring at first. You may miss the "action" associated with getting or using chemicals even more than you miss alcohol or drugs.

You will need to replace drug and alcohol activities with new ones so that boredom is not an excuse to use chemicals again. Perhaps, like many others, you gave up some of your nondrug and alcohol interests over time as your addiction took over your life.

You may also feel bored with your job, your relationships, or other life circumstances. Chemical use may have covered up your boredom and unhappiness in these areas. Try to figure out why you are bored with your life if this is the case with you. For example, maybe you are bored in your primary relationship because your needs aren't getting met. Perhaps you are bored at work because you aren't able to use your talents or your job isn't challenging.

Answer the following questions to assess where you stand in relation to boredom and to more clearly see how your addiction may have contributed to it:

1. On a scale of 1 to 10, how much of a problem is your boredom or how you cope with it (✓ your rating).

1	*3*	*5*	*7*	*10*
No	*Moderate*	*Significant*	*Serious*	*Severe*
Problem	*Problem*	*Problem*	*Problem*	*Problem*

_____   _____   _____   _____   _____

If you wrote down a rating of three or more, it is recommended that you learn new ways of dealing with boredom. If you wrote down a rating of five or more, it is recommended that you consider therapy if you are not already in treatment.

2. I enjoy the following hobbies or activities:

_____

_____

_____

3.   As a result of my chemical dependency, I gave up these activities:

_____

_____

_____

_____

4.   I would like to get involved in these activities again:

_____

_____

_____

_____

5.   New activities or interests that I would like to get involved in include:

_____

_____

_____

_____

6.   I (am or am not) bored and in need of a lot of "action" or excitement. Explain your answer.

_____

_____

_____

_____

7.   What excites me and makes me feel good about life is:

_____

_____

_____

_____

_____

Setting a Goal

My *Goal* in relation to my boredom is:

_____

_____

Steps **I will take to reach this goal are:**

_____

_____

_____

Potential benefits **of reaching my goal are:**

_____

_____

_____

Boredom Busters

- *Regain lost activities.*

  Try to regain "lost" activities that you enjoyed before your addiction took over your life. Make sure these are not activities you associate with using alcohol or other drugs, or that threaten your ongoing recovery.

- *Develop new leisure interests.*

  Learn new hobbies, develop new interests, or find new forms of pleasure or enjoyment. Recovery gives you an opportunity to expand your horizons and try new activities. Think of something you always wanted to do but never quite got around to doing, and try it. There really are endless activities or hobbies you could get involved in. Find those that interest you and do them! Don't allow yourself to make excuses why you can't do these activities.

- *Build structure into your daily life.*

  The more structured your life, especially in the early months of recovery, the less time you have to feel bored. When structuring your time, make sure you build fun and relaxation into your day-to-day life so it isn't only focused on work, responsibilities, or recovery. Find a balance in leisure activities involving other people and those involving just yourself. While it's good to socialize with others and share mutual interests and activities, it is also good to have things to do that you can enjoy while you are alone.

- *Know your high-risk times for boredom.*

  Identify high-risk times for feeling bored and plan activities as needed during these times. For most people in recovery, weekends and evenings are the toughest, especially at first. Your high-risk times are when you need the most structure in your life. Force yourself if you have to in order to get active in social situations or activities. Many people have a good time and enjoy themselves in situations they initially dreaded or had to force themselves to attend.

- *Participate in social activities sponsored by 12-Step groups or recovery clubs.*

  Many 12 Step groups sponsor social or recreational activities. Likewise, recovery clubs offer a sober atmosphere in which to relate to others and participate in social events such as dances or dinners.

- *Think differently about boredom.*

Change your attitudes and beliefs about boredom. For example, expect some boredom in your life and don't expect to have a life filled with enjoyable activities. Even though it helps for you to structure your time, don't think you always have to be busy at something every hour of every day, especially fun activities. It's OK to have time for yourself that isn't planned. Remember, if you feel bored it is *your* problem, not someone else's. Keep reminding yourself you can find things to break your boredom.

- *Focus on enjoying the simple things in life.*

If you have a need for high levels of action, excitement, and risk, try to learn how to enjoy the simple, day-to-day pleasures life can offer. Don't expect to always be able to satisfy your need for action or excitement. Life simply doesn't work that way.

- *Improve relationships and initiate activities with others.*

Focus your attention on nurturing and improving your personal relationships. Find new people to develop relationships with if needed. Being involved in positive relationships adds richness to your life, especially if you share mutual interests or activities with others. If you feel bored or lonely and want to be with other people, be assertive and take the initiative. Call others and invite them out to share a mutual interest. Don't wait for others to take the initiative. Pick up the phone and get the ball rolling. When doing this, consider the interests of others as well as your own. Don't expect to always do what you want. Instead, learn to enjoy what others like to do. On the other hand, make sure you spend time doing things that are fun and enjoyable to you.

- *Go slow in making major life changes.*

Carefully evaluate relationship or job boredom before making any major changes. Don't make quick or impulsive changes, especially if they are major ones. For example, if you are bored with work, you should figure out why. But before you make any change, closely examine the potential risk and benefits. The same holds true with a personal relationship. If you are bored with your spouse, partner, or mate, figure out why and how to make things better before you decide to end the relationship.

- *Use therapy to help you with feelings of emptiness.*

If you feel empty inside and nothing has meaning or purpose in your life, consult a professional mental health therapist. You may benefit from therapy. A severe feeling of emptiness sometimes is a symptom of a psychiatric illness such as depression or a personality problem.

SESSION 17
Coping with Depression

Many people with alcohol and drug problems also experience depression. Drugs such as alcohol, opiates, tranquilizers, and sedatives depress the central nervous system and can cause you to feel depressed. Depression is also associated with "crashing" from the effects of cocaine or other stimulant drugs.

Problems and losses caused by chemical dependency can cause feelings of depression. Relationships, jobs, status, health, money, dignity, and self-esteem are frequently lost as a result of addiction.

Depression can also be caused by a relapse to chemical use. This is especially true after a significant period of abstinence from chemicals.

For many, simply getting and staying sober or clean helps decrease or eliminate feelings of depression. This is not true for everyone, however. Some still feel depressed even after being sober or clean for weeks or months. Yet others experience depression long after getting sober or clean from chemicals.

Some people have a type of clinical depression that is more than the blues or feeling down that everyone feels from time to time. This condition is referred to as *major depression* and requires professional treatment. Chemically dependent people have higher rates of major depression than the general population.

Major depression involves experiencing many symptoms nearly every day, for two weeks or longer. These symptoms include: feeling depressed; being unable to experience pleasure; loss of appetite; decrease in sexual desire or energy; difficulty concentrating; significant weight change; problems falling asleep, staying asleep, or sleeping too much; feeling agitated or restless; feeling hopeless, helpless, worthless, or guilty; or even feeling like life is not worth living or making an actual attempt at suicide. For some, depressive symptoms have been more or less present for months and months, or even longer.

Even if you don't have depressive illness you can benefit from learning new ways to handle feelings of depression so that your recovery goes better. Beginning on the next page are some questions to help you assess your depression.

1. I have experienced the following symptoms for this long: (Use a 10-point scale when determining "to what degree" you are experiencing a specific symptom with 1=not at all; 5=to a significant degree; 10=to a serious degree).

Symptom	To What Degree? (1-10)	How Long
Feeling depressed or sad		
Trouble experiencing pleasure		
Appetite disturbance		
Sleep disturbance		
Feeling agitated or irritable		
Feeling slowed down		
Difficulty concentrating or remembering things		
Feeling helpless, hopeless, or guilty		
Loss or decrease in sexual desire		
Thoughts of taking life		
Plan to take your life		
Actual suicide attempt		

2. On a scale of 1 to 10, how much of a problem is depression for you (√ your rating)?

1	3	5	7	10
No Problem	Moderate Problem	Significant Problem	Serious Problem	Severe Problem

_____   _____   _____   _____   _____

If your rating was three or higher, you should consider talking with a professional to determine if you need treatment. If your rating was five or higher, you should definitely seek professional help. If you have strong thoughts of taking your life, an actual plan, or have made an attempt, call a mental health professional now if you aren't already in treatment.

3. Depression has affected my life in the following ways:

_____

_____

_____

_____

4. I am currently depressed because:

_____

_____

_____

_____

5. I tend to have a lot of negative, pessimistic, or depressing thoughts about myself or the future.

____ Yes   ____ No

Explain your answer.

_____

_____

_____

_____

6. My use of alcohol or drugs and my depression are connected in the following ways:

_____

_____

Setting a Goal

My *Goal* in relation to my depression is:

_____

_____

Steps I will take to reach this goal are:

_____

_____

_____

_____

Potential benefits of reaching my goal are:

_____

_____

_____

_____

Coping with Depression

- *Find out the problems that are causing you to feel depressed and do something about them.*

Solving problems contributing to depression should help you feel better. If you feel depressed because you are overweight, then do something about your weight. If you feel depressed because you hate your job, look at other options. If you feel depressed because your relationships are unsatisfying, look for ways to improve these relationships or develop new ones. However, depression is not always related to "problems" or "life events." Sometimes, biological factors may be the primary factor contributing to depression. This is especially true of people who have two or more episodes of clinical depression. This is called **recurrent depression**, and having this type of depression increases your chances of having future episodes. Make sure you get a thorough physical examination so that medical causes of depression can be ruled-out first.

Read recovery literature such as *Learning to Live Again, Passages Through Recovery, The Relapse/Recovery Grid, Understanding Addictive Disease*, and others listed in the Appendix.

- *Evaluate your relationships with other people.*

  Develop new relationships or improve relationships that are problematic and which contribute to your feeling depressed. Look at whether your emotional needs are getting satisfied from your current relationships.

- *Make amends.*

  Depression can be connected to guilt associated with hurting others because of your chemical dependency. Making amends can help you feel less depressed and better about yourself. The AA/NA 12-Step program can help guide you through the process of making amends. A counselor or sponsor can help you determine when you are ready to make amends to specific individuals you feel were hurt by your chemical use.

- *Keep active.*

  Even if you have to force yourself to do things, keep active in your social relationhips and with your hobbies and interests. When you least want to do things may be when you most need to. Physical activity like walking, running, working out, working around the house or yard, or playing sports may indirectly help improve your depression.

- *Talk about your feelings and problems with others.*

  Share your feelings of sadness or depression with supportive people such as close friends or family members. Talk about your feelings with your sponsor or a counselor. Venting feelings may provide you with some relief and help you gain a different perspective on your depression. Or you may learn some new ideas on coping with depression from other people. However, you must guard against always talking about your feelings with others. People usually are supportive to a degree. If you don't try to help yourself and do some things differently to cope with your depression, others can get tired of hearing you constantly talk about your depressed feelings.

- *Look for other emotions or feelings that may contribute to, or be associated with, depression.*

  Other emotions may contribute to feelings of depression. Some people are prone to feeling more depressed when they suppress or hold on to feelings of anger. Others who feel guilty and shameful may be prone to depression if they don't figure out ways to work through these feelings. Some people get depressed as a result of constantly feeling anxious or fearful.

- *Change your depressed thoughts.*

  Your thoughts can contribute to feelings of depression. Learn to identify and challenge negative, pessimistic, or depressed thoughts. Avoid making mountains out of molehills, always looking at the negative side of things, always expecting the worse-case scenario, or dwelling on your mistakes or shortcomings. You can use self-talk strategies to change negative thoughts (for example, in response to making a mistake, instead of saying, "I'm not capable of doing this," say, "I made a mistake. It's no big deal, everyone makes mistakes").

- *Focus on positive things.*

  Make sure you acknowledge your positive points or strengths. Don't take yourself for granted, and give yourself credit for your positive qualities. Take an inventory of your achievements or the positive things happening in your life, no matter how small. Learn to look at the "other" side of things when you catch yourself thinking negatively. For example, suppose you lost twenty-five pounds over several months only to gain five back. Rather than put yourself down and feel depressed for gaining five pounds back, remind yourself that you still are twenty pounds down from your previous weight. Remember, sometimes it's not so much what you do but how you think about what you do that determines how you feel.

- *Keep a journal.*

  Writing about your feelings can help you release them or better understand them. This can also help you to figure out if there are patterns to your feelings and behaviors. For example, suppose you discover that you always tend to feel more depressed after visiting your parents. In exploring this further, you discover these feelings relate to constantly being criticized by your father, or because your mother usually is drunk when you visit and this triggers bad feelings and memories from the past. A journal can also help you keep track of changes in your depression over time as well as the positive coping strategies that seem to help you the most. In addition, you can write about positive or hopeful things that happen to you each day.

- *Participate in pleasant activities each day.*

  Put some time aside each day to do something that is fun, enjoyable, or pleasurable. It doesn't matter how small this is. Even small things like taking fifteen minutes to yourself each day to read a magazine and enjoy a cup of coffee or tea may help you feel better.

- *Identify and plan future activities that you can look forward to enjoying.*

  We all need things to look forward to, whether it is buying something nice for ourselves, taking a vacation, or participating in an enjoyable activity. Having things to look forward to breaks up the monotony of doing the same old things over and over. It provides a focus for your energy and can make you feel invested in life. Set some goals in relation to activities, events, or experiences that you can plan and look forward to.

- *If your depression doesn't get better, seek an evaluation by a mental health professional.*

  If these or other coping techniques don't seem to help much, and your depression continues and causes you personal suffering or interferes with your life, seek an evaluation with a mental health professional. There are many different types of treatment that are effective for clinical depression. These include various types of therapy as well as the use of antidepressant medications. Not all clinical depressions need medications. But if yours does, you should not feel guilty. It is not the same as drinking alcohol or using drugs to get high or loaded.

  For many people, clinical depression is a lifelong disorder requiring ongoing treatment. If you have had two or more episodes of serious depression you probably need ongoing treatment, even after your depression improves or lifts completely. People who stop treatment for depression put themselves at risk for relapse in the future.

SECTION V

Building Relationships
and
Support

SESSION 18
Your Family and Recovery

Families are often affected by a member's dual disorders. Mood or atmosphere, communication, how members get along, and financial condition are just a few examples of the areas of family life that are affected. In addition, the physical, emotional, and spiritual health of individual members can also be affected. An important aspect of your recovery is to understand how your family was actually affected by your dual disorders and to encourage them to get involved in recovery if needed.

Some of the common concerns and questions of families include the following:

- *Diagnosis and causes of illness* — families want to know what your disorders are and what caused them.

- *Treatment* — family members want to know how long you might have to be in treatment, how it can help you, and what should be done if treatment doesn't appear to work.

- *Medications* — families are often concerned with how long you will have to take medicines, what side effects you may experience, and what may happen if you drink alcohol or use illicit drugs when you're on medications for a psychiatric disorder.

- *Responsibility* — families are often concerned about where their responsibility ends and yours begins in relation to your recovery. Sometimes families worry about doing too much for you and taking over too many of your responsibilities.

- *Family role in treatment* — families wonder to what degree they should get involved in your treatment. Some worry about getting blamed for your problems. Members also wonder whether they need help themselves in order to cope with their reactions and feelings.

- *Other family members getting sick* — with psychiatric illness in particular, families are often concerned that if one member has an illness another person may get sick as well. As I've said before, many psychiatric illnesses and chemical dependencies run in families, making members more vulnerable to getting one or more of these disorders.

- *Threat of loss* — family members often worry they may lose the member with dual disorders, particularly when this person is a parent. They sometimes also feel deprived of their time, attention, and love as well. This is especially true in cases where the disorder is so severe you just cannot be emotionally available to your family or you are unable to take care of them.

- *Threat to security* — family members often worry about their physical, emotional, and psychological security, especially when a parent is the one with dual disorders. If your behaviors include violence or very poor judgment in which you do things to threaten the security of your family, they are likely to feel even more insecure.

- *Long-term outcome* — another typical concern of families relates to the worry they have about the long-term outcome of treatment. They wonder how your illness and participation in recovery may affect you in the long term. Again, this is particularly true in families where the member with dual disorders has been in the hospital many times or has had serious life problems as a result of the psychiatric and addiction problems.

- *Financial burden* — the cost of treatment, expenses associated with the legal system, and loss of income related to being able to keep a job or find a job often can create a financial burden on the family. If, as a parent, your alcohol or drug use or your psychiatric symptoms led to you being unable to work and provide for your family, financial problems probably occurred.

- *Emotional burden* — families often feel emotionally drained, tired, or burned-out from dealing with dual disorders and related behaviors. In some cases they may have symptoms of psychiatric illness themselves, such as a serious mood disorder or anxiety disorder. Or family members may have their own alcohol or drug problems.

- *Effectiveness of treatment* — families often worry whether treatment will be able to help you. Because relapse rates are high with chronic psychiatric illness as well as addiction, families wonder if treatment will be helpful in your case. If you have been in multiple treatments and have been on a number of different medications over the years and you still show a lot of symptoms, your family is even more likely to have concerns about whether treatment can help you.

- *Lack of motivation to get well* — because many people with dual disorders don't acknowledge their problems or seek help on their own, families often worry about how to encourage their ill member to get help. Once the dual diagnosis member is in treatment, families often worry about how to deal with any lack of motivation their member may have to work their recovery program and make positive changes.

- *Suicide* — suicide attempts and threats are often very stressful to families. Families worry about whether they can detect suicidal thinking and do anything about it.

- *Relapse of psychiatric illness* — another concern is whether you'll get sick again with the symptoms of your psychiatric illness. If you've had multiple episodes of illness over time or a chronic course of illness, families often worry about your symptoms coming back or getting worse.

- *Alcohol or drug relapse* — because alcohol and drugs cause so many problems within the family, members often worry whether you'll pick up and use again. This is particularly true if you've been in recovery before and have relapsed several times.

- *Hospitalization* — families worry if hospitalization is needed in certain cases where your symptoms return or your alcohol or drug use gets out of control. Families are particularly concerned about how to get you into the hospital when you resist and refuse to go along with their recommendations to get help in the hospital. If your behavior is a serious threat to yourself or others and they have to hospitalize you involuntarily, families often feel guilty for doing this.

As much as possible, try to put yourself in your family's shoes. If you can understand what it has been like from their point of view to cope with your alcohol and drug use and your psychiatric disorder, this may lead you to a greater understanding of their experiences. The more you and your family can understand each other, the better it is for everyone involved.

Describe below how you think your family has been affected by your dual disorders:

Your family unit:

_____

_____

_____

_____

Your spouse/partner:

_____

_____

_____

_____

Your children/stepchildren:

_____

_____

_____

_____

Other family members (parents, siblings, etc.):

_____

_____

_____

_____

Have any of your family members expressed their concerns about your alcohol or other drug use or your psychiatric condition? If yes, what did they tell you?

_____

_____

_____

_____

At some point in your recovery, you should consider making amends to your family for the difficulties caused by your dual disorders. Who, when, and how to do this are important considerations that you should first discuss with your doctor, therapist, or AA/NA sponsor. While you don't want to rush into this too quickly, you also must guard against putting it off indefinitely.

You can begin this process by getting your family involved in recovery if possible and by making sure you spend time with them. It is helpful to sit down and talk face-to-face with family members and hear straight from them what it was like and how they felt about both your addiction and your psychiatric disorder. However, since not all family members are able, willing, or even should be involved in recovery, this is an issue that you should discuss first with your therapist or sponsor. He or she can help you determine what to do about this issue. There are instances where the harm has been so great that directly making amends to a family member is not advised. Participating in family therapy is often helpful in addressing some of these important issues in recovery.

Nicole's Effect on Her Family and Her Plan

My depression, hurting myself and threatening suicide too many times to count, and abuse of alcohol and drugs has really hurt my parents a lot. I've done about everything to my parents that you could imagine one could do including lying to them, threatening to hurt myself, getting high and saying nasty things to their face, and basically just being rotten to them. Since I've been in and out of psych hospitals and rehab programs, outpatient counseling and AA and NA too many times to count, I know that my words to them will be shallow if they are not backed up with a plan. Frankly, I know they're probably tired of me making verbal amends to them only to go out and do the same things over and over.

I guess you could say it's been an emotional and a financial strain on my parents. And my sister, she basically has washed her hands of me. I've said a lot of bad things to her as well as stormed over to her apartment on many occasions when I've either been high or upset with someone.

It's not going to be easy, but I know what I have to do to get closer to my family. The first and most important thing is that I have to stay in treatment. I have to stay on my medication, go to therapy and not miss appointments, and go to my NA meetings. There's no ifs, ands, or buts about any of this. I also have talked to my doctor and my outpatient therapist and we have agreed that I'm going to bring my parents to sessions every month. This way we can talk about my progress as well as any problems I'm having. We can also talk about what's realistic for them in terms of how they can help me as well as what I need to do myself.

My parents have always stood beside me and probably have done too much for me in the past. In some ways I guess you could say that they have to get a little tougher on me. The bottom line is that if we work together, there is a greater chance that I can do better in my recovery and improve things with my family.

Your Children

Sometimes, children in families in which a parent has a psychiatric disorder, alcohol or drug abuse problem, or both develop serious problems themselves. These may be emotional, behavioral, school, or alcohol and drug problems. If you have children and one or more of them shows any of the following, arrange to have them evaluated by a mental health professional to determine if special treatment is needed:

- severe anxiety
- depression or mood swings
- hears voices or has very bizarre thoughts (for example, that people are trying to put thoughts in or take them out of their heads)
- becomes violent with other people
- expresses thoughts of suicide
- has trouble concentrating or completing schoolwork, leading to poor grades
- skips school a lot
- has trouble getting along with other kids at home or school
- has trouble with the law

If any of your children are using alcohol or drugs, arrange to have them treated by a drug or alcohol treatment professional.

Children benefit from participating in support groups such as Alateen or treatment sessions with a therapist. If you have any concerns about how your children may have been affected by your dual disorders, ask your social worker or other members of your treatment team what services may be available for them. When children learn about dual disorders, it helps them better understand what their parent has gone through.

In your opinion, do any of your children need an evaluation for a possible mental health problem or alcohol/drug use problem?

_____ Yes   _____ No

If you answered yes, what steps can you take to get your child an assessment and/or treatment?

_____

_____

_____

Daryl's Effects on His Son and His Plan

I know my addiction and my crazy behavior really messed up my family. My nine-year-old son, Daryl, Jr., is having a lot of trouble. He gets in fights all the time at school, sasses the teacher, and doesn't do what he is told. He has trouble getting along with his brothers and sisters, too. Daryl even sasses me and doesn't listen to me sometimes. Things seem to be getting worse instead of better. Even though I'm doing better and I'm in recovery now, Daryl is still having trouble. So me and my wife decided that we need to get him seen to figure out if he needs treatment, too. I talked this over with my outpatient therapist and we made an arrangement for him to get an evaluation and for the family to be seen as well. This way we can figure out if any kind of treatment will be needed for Daryl. Ain't no doubt in my mind that the boy needs help. This is the time to do it now.

Setting a Goal

My *Goal* in relation to my children or family is:

_____

_____

Steps I will take to reach this goal are:

_____

_____

_____

Potential benefits of reaching my goal are:

_____

_____

_____

SESSION 19
Saying No to Getting High

One of the biggest factors contributing to relapse to alcohol or drug use is pressure from other people to use chemicals. Pressures may be direct in which other people offer you chemicals or invite you to use with them or party. Pressures may also be indirect and occur when you're in situations where other people are using but they aren't asking you directly to use chemicals with them. Office parties, graduations, weddings, and other social events are just some activities where people may be drinking alcohol and not offering any to you directly. By thinking ahead and identifying the social pressures you are likely to experience in figuring out some way to refuse offers to get high, you put yourself in a better position to keep your sobriety.

When you're in a situation where you feel direct or indirect pressure to use chemicals, sometimes it taps a part of you that still wants to get high. As a result, you may feel anxious, worried, or even excited. It is not unusual to have mixed feelings where part of you wants to give in to the pressure to use and part of you doesn't want to give in. Remember, even though you may *want* to use doesn't mean you *have* to use. Therefore, you have to be prepared with some ways to say no to drugs or alcohol and get out of situations in which you experience very strong pressure to get high.

You also need to be able to identify people that you have a relationship with who pose a threat to your ongoing sobriety. These are people who want to get high with you or who want to use while they're around you. For example, if you are trying to stay clean from cocaine or alcohol and your partner or spouse gets high in the apartment or at your home, this increases your risk for relapse. It's simply just too hard to stay straight when other people around you are getting high in front of you. If your close relationships involve people who get high and have a drug or alcohol problem, you're going to have to figure out ways of coping with this in order to protect your own recovery. This is something you should talk over with your therapist, doctor, and sponsor in self-help programs.

Answer the following questions to help you develop your plan to not give in to pressures to use alcohol or drugs:

1. List people who are likely to directly invite you to use alcohol or drugs or likely to use while they are around you and make you feel pressure to get high.

_____   _____

_____   _____

_____   _____

_____   _____

2. Imagine that you're being offered alcohol or drugs right now. Write down the *feelings* this often triggers in you.

    Example: "I feel tempted but scared."

    _____

    _____

    _____

    _____

    Write down the *thoughts* that this triggers.

    Example: "Man, I'd really like to fit in and get high but I know it ain't the best thing for me."

    _____

    _____

    _____

    _____

3. Imagine you're offered your drug of choice by one of the people listed in question #1. State at least 3 strategies you could use to refuse this offer and protect your sobriety.

    Example: "I'll just say straight out that I'm in recovery and I'm not using and don't offer me anything again."

    _____

    _____

    _____

    _____

4. If you imagine yourself giving in to the social pressure to use alcohol or other drugs, how is this likely to affect you?

    Example: "I'll feel disappointed in myself and angry because I know after the high wears off, I'll realize it just wasn't worth it."

    _____

    _____

    _____

    _____

5. Imagine yourself successfully refusing the offer to get high, and state how this will affect you as well.

Example: "I'll feel good about myself for making the right decision to stay clean."

_____

_____

_____

_____

Strategies to Cope with Pressures to Get High

1. State straight out that you don't want to use alcohol or drugs.

2. Tell the person offering that you're in recovery and you would appreciate it if they didn't offer you alcohol or drugs again.

3. Tell the person that you're on medication and you can't drink or use anything while you're on medication.

4. Get out of the situation as quickly as you can if you're feeling increasing pressure to use.

5. If there is an upcoming event where you may feel pressure to use, such as a graduation party or wedding that you don't want to miss, take a support person with you—a friend in recovery, sponsor, or family member—who knows about your recovery.

Coping with Pressures to Stop Taking Your Medicine

Some people in recovery will be told by others in recovery to stop taking medication. You may be made to feel guilty or led to believe that taking medication for a psychiatric disorder means that you're not sober or clean as part of your recovery. Don't believe this for a minute, because taking medication for a psychiatric illness does not mean that you're not in recovery. In fact, not taking the medication is more likely to increase your risk of relapse. Remember, other people cannot play doctor and if you're on medication for a specific psychiatric illness then you need to continue to take it. If any person tries to convince you to get off your medication, don't give in to this pressure.

Many have found it helpful to think about this ahead of time and devise some ways they would cope with pressures to get off medication. In the space below write two or more examples of how you could respond if another person tells you to quit taking your medication.

_____

_____

_____

_____

_____

_____

SESSION 20
Developing and Using a Relapse Prevention Support System

No one can recover alone. It is important to develop and use a support system as part of your recovery. A relapse prevention support system consists of people in your life who can help you and support your recovery. These are people you can lean on during rough times or who are important in your day-to-day life.

Your support system usually involves the following: professionals who provide your treatment; AA, NA, or dual recovery support group sponsors or members; close friends; and family members. These should be people with whom you have regular contact and can share your thoughts, feelings, and struggles. People in your network ideally are those who also are willing to be honest with you and tell you if you are slacking off your recovery program or acting in ways that increase the chances of a relapse. People in your recovery network should be ones who will help you if you relapse to your psychiatric illness or your addiction.

You can use this network in many ways: for emotional support, to discuss a problem, to discuss thoughts about dropping out of treatment, to talk through strong desires to use alcohol or drugs, or to share some time together in a social or recreational activity. Regular discussions with members of your network such as a sponsor or counselor can help you identify problems early and figure out plans to deal with these before a relapse occurs.

Sometimes other people will notice relapse warning signs before you do. You may find it helpful to ask members of your support network to point out any warning signs they notice. Keep in mind, however, that it is your responsibility to take action to cope with your warning signs if someone points them out.

Individuals who have a solid support system are more likely than others to maintain their recovery. They are more likely to feel secure because of having a network of people they can rely on to support efforts at recovery and help with problems.

Once again, it is important to read widely in the available recovery literature. Begin with *Learning to Live Again* and others from the Appendix at the end of this workbook.

Recovery Activity

1. List the names and phone numbers of five people you can rely on for support and help in recovering from dual disorders:

   (1) _____

   (2) _____

   (3) _____

   (4) _____

   (5) _____

2. Do you have a sponsor in AA, NA, or dual recovery group? ___ Yes ___ No
   If no, how could a sponsor help you?

   _____

   _____

   _____

3. List five benefits of having a relapse prevention support network.

   (1) _____

   (2) _____

   (3) _____

   (4) _____

   (5) _____

4. List five ways that members of your relapse prevention support network could be of help to you in your recovery.

   (1) _____

   (2) _____

   (3) _____

   (4) _____

   (5) _____

5. Why is it important to have a relapse prevention support network?

   _____

   _____

   _____

AA/NA/DRA, Mental Health Support Groups, and Recovery Clubs

Involvement in self-help recovery programs offers you many benefits. Your recovery from dual disorders will go better if you take advantage of various support programs available in your community. Your treatment team can help you figure out which of the following can help you stay clean or sober and help you in your recovery from psychiatric illness:

- attending AA/NA, Dual Recovery Anonymous (DRA), or mental health support groups
- working the 12-Step program of AA/NA/DRA
- getting a sponsor to help you use the "tools" of recovery
- reading recovery literature
- spending time at "recovery clubs"

AA/NA/DRA Meetings

AA, NA, and DRA offer an important source of ongoing support for recovery from alcohol and drug abuse disorders. There are different kinds of meetings. One kind is called a "lead meeting" that involves a person sharing his or her story of addiction and recovery. Another kind of meeting is called a "discussion meeting" and allows all present to share their ideas and experiences related to the topic under discussion. Some meetings are "closed" and are available only to those with alcohol or drug problems. Others are "open" and can be attended by anyone. There are many meetings for "special" groups of people such as business people, health care professionals, gay men or lesbian women, young people, newcomers, etc. By checking around and attending different meetings, you should be able to find some that you feel can help you.

Some AA/NA meetings are specifically designated for people with dual disorders. These "dual recovery" meetings provide a chance to talk about both your psychiatric illness and your alcohol/drug abuse. Recovery meetings that focus on dual disorders go by a lot of different names. Some examples include: double trouble, MISA, CAMI, SAMI, and dual recovery. While many people with dual disorders feel that traditional AA/NA meetings benefit them, others prefer going to these special meetings as well, or to DRA meetings.

The 12 Steps of AA/NA/DRA

The 12-Step program of AA/NA/DRA offers an excellent mechanism to make positive changes and stay clean or sober. The 12-Step program offers you the opportunity to work on changing yourself.

Other Support Groups for Addiction

Some communities have other types of support groups to help in recovery from alcohol or drug problems. Some local support programs that you may wish to learn more about to determine if they can help you include Women for Sobriety (WFS) and Rational Recovery (RR). Ask your treatment team for more information.

Mental Health Support Groups

Support groups are also available for people with mental health problems such as depression, bipolar disorder, schizophrenia, and other disorders. These groups provide a chance to learn about mental health problems and recovery from them. Similar to AA/NA/ DRA meetings, people share hope, strength, and experience and help each other out.

Family Support Groups

There are many self-help support groups available for families as well. These include groups such as AlAnon or NarAnon that relate specifically to coping with alcohol and drug abuse in the family and groups related to psychiatric illness and the family. If your family is involved in your treatment, we highly recommend that family support groups be used. By attending meetings, families learn about illness, recovery, and how they can cope with their own feelings. Family groups provide families with a chance to get support from others and discuss their own concerns.

Sponsorship

An extremely helpful aspect of self-help programs is sponsorship. A "sponsor" is a person in a self-help program who has established a solid period of recovery (usually a couple of years or longer). A sponsor helps newcomers learn to use the "tools" of recovery. A sponsor can help in many ways: attending meetings with you, being available for daily discussions on the phone, helping you work the 12 Steps, and being there for you during difficult times.

You can get a sponsor in several ways: ask a member at a meeting whom you know has some good recovery time to sponsor you; ask the chairperson at a meeting to help you find a sponsor; call AA/NA/DRA and ask if they can help you get a sponsor; or ask a staff member to help you find a sponsor.

Recovery Literature

There is a lot of information available to help you better understand addiction, mental health, dual disorders, and recovery. This includes pamphlets, workbooks, books, audiotapes, and videotapes. Ask your primary therapist, another member of your treatment team, or your sponsor for specific recommendations. Some of the written materials were developed by people like yourself who are recovering from an addiction, mental health, or dual disorders. Other materials were developed by professionals on the following topics: AA, NA, sponsorship, the 12 Steps, depression, anxiety, anger, psychiatric illness, relapse, relapse prevention, addiction, cocaine, alcohol and other drugs, family recovery, and other topics. See the Appendix at the end of this workbook for a beginning list.

Recovery Clubs

Recovery is a process that takes time. The weeks and months after rehab or inpatient treatment is a critical time period in recovery. It is suggested that you fill your time with positive, constructive activities to replace time previously spent using chemicals. Also, avoid negative people, places, and things that trigger a desire to get high and hinder your recovery program.

The idea of recovery clubs came about as a way of helping fill time in a constructive way. All basically have the same purpose for you as a recovering addict or alcoholic. The purpose is to provide a safe environment in which you can meet and talk with other recovering people, attend meetings, and share ideas about the process of recovery. Most recovery clubs have recreational activities such as pool tables, ping pong tables, and places where one can play cards. While doing these activities, you are in a constructive atmosphere that promotes openness and honesty, which is important not only in the beginning stages of recovery but should be learned in order to continue a good or healthy program of recovery.

The hours of operation vary from club to club, but usually the hours are from early morning until late at night if not beyond midnight on weekends. Many clubs sponsor dances, picnics, and periodic large social events that are attended by many people from support groups such as AA, NA, DRA, Alanon, Adult Children, CA, and GA.

Food is also available at nominal cost for the people attending recovery clubs. The quality of food is not gourmet by any standard, but it is very moderately priced and provides a place where you can go to have breakfast, lunch, or dinner in a safe environment where there are no chemicals.

Recovery Planning Task

1.   Check the following types of support groups that you participate in:

        ____   AA meetings
        ____   NA meetings
        ____   DRA or other types of dual recovery meetings
        ____   Mental health support group meetings

113

2.   List three ways that you think these support groups can help you:

      (1) _____
      (2) _____
      (3) _____

3.   List three benefits of working the 12-Step program of AA/NA/DRA:

      (1) _____
      (2) _____
      (3) _____

4.   List three ways a sponsor can help you:

      (1) _____
      (2) _____
      (3) _____

5.   If you do not already have a sponsor, do you plan to get one? If yes, when? If no, why not?

      _____
      _____
      _____

6.   List three benefits of reading recovery literature on a regular basis:

      (1) _____
      (2) _____
      (3) _____

7.   List three benefits of spending time in a recovery club:

      (1) _____
      (2) _____
      (3) _____

Step 1 Worksheet

1.   In your own words, state what you think Step 1 means:

_____

_____

_____

_____

_____

2.   Give some examples of your own powerlessness over alcohol or drugs:

(1) _____

(2) _____

(3) _____

(4) _____

(5) _____

(6) _____

3.   Give some examples of how your alcohol and drug use led to unmanageability in your life:

(1) _____

(2) _____

(3) _____

(4) _____

(5) _____

(6) _____

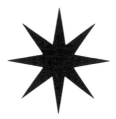

SECTION VI

Changing the Self: A Holistic Approach

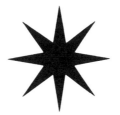

SESSION 22
Changing Self-defeating and Self-destructive Behaviors

Self-destructive behaviors refer to involvement in activities that threaten serious harm to yourself. These behaviors can also pose a threat to your family, relationships, and job as well as your physical, emotional, spiritual, or financial well-being. These include addictive behaviors such as chemical dependency, compulsive gambling, overeating, or sex.

Self-destructive behaviors also include actual attempts to hurt yourself or take your own life through a suicidal gesture. These behaviors include putting yourself in danger by driving a car recklessly, engaging in other risky behaviors, acting aggressively or violently toward other people, getting into fights, or setting up situations with others in which the likelihood of a violent episode will occur.

Self-defeating behaviors are those behaviors that hurt your emotional well-being or your relationships. Patterns of self-defeating behavior can show in the way you relate to other people, cope with problems or stress, or deal with taking care of your basic needs. Examples of self-defeating patterns of behavior include jumping from one relationship to the next, getting easily bored and leaving your partner, getting involved in relationships with people who do not take care of your needs and are abusive to you, or getting into a relationship in which you have very little in common with the other person and are very likely to become dissatisfied with this person. Sometimes these self-defeating patterns are very obvious. Other times they are less obvious and you have to look very closely at your life to figure out whether or not they are present.

Here are some common examples of self-destructive and self-defeating behaviors. Place a ✓ next to the ones that apply to you.

_____ Being overly controlling with others.

_____ Jumping from one relationship to the next.

_____ Getting easily bored with my partner.

_____ Moving in with a partner who I have known for only a short period of time.

_____ Purposely saying things that hurt other people.

_____ Holding my feelings inside and not communicating directly to other people who are important to me such as a partner or family member.

_____ Letting people take advantage of me and holding on to my resentments.

____ Picking up strangers or people I don't know very well and having sex with them.

____ Not using protection when having sex.

____ Getting involved too quickly in a romantic relationship.

____ Not spending time with my children or family members in order to keep the relationships active.

____ Getting involved in relationships that are physically or emotionally abusive.

____ Using intimidation and anger to keep people on their guard so they can't get close to me.

____ Conning others and scamming to get money, or taking advantage of them in other ways.

____ Hanging out with other people who are getting high on alcohol or drugs and thinking that I will be able to do this and not be tempted to use myself.

____ Getting into fights or hurting other people through violence.

____ Quitting jobs impulsively.

____ Not being responsible on the job (coming in late, leaving early, missing a lot of work, arguing with co-workers, or not performing my duties as I should).

____ Managing my money very poorly and getting myself deep in debt.

____ Spending money I need for basic necessities on things that I don't need.

____ Starting things and not finishing them (starting a project and not finishing it, starting a school or vocational project and not finishing, or setting some other goal that I begin to work toward and just forget about and stop working toward achieving this goal).

____ Not setting any goals or having any sense of direction in your life.

____ Making mistakes and not accepting responsibility for my actions but rather blaming bad fortune or other people for my mistakes or misfortunes.

____ Not having any structure or routine built into my life so that I have a sense of regularity and a sense of direction.

_____ Not following through with my medical treatment or medical advice regarding physical problems.

_____ Not following through with treatment or advice from my doctor or therapist regarding ways to help myself with my psychiatric or drug and alcohol problem.

_____ Not being open-minded regarding feedback given to me by an NA, AA, or CA sponsor or other members of 12-Step programs.

_____ Not taking suggestions provided to me by members of mental health support groups or dual recovery support groups.

_____ Getting high on alcohol or other drugs.

_____ Gambling too much or compulsively.

_____ Overeating.

_____ Eating and then making myself vomit.

_____ Compulsive sexual behavior.

_____ Cutting, burning, or damaging my body.

_____ Getting tatoos all over my body.

_____ Keeping alcohol or drugs in my home in order to test myself.

_____ Spending too much time watching TV.

_____ Spending too much idle time goofing off.

_____ Getting involved in too many projects or activities.

_____ Spending too much time working at the expense of having time to spend with family or friends, or engage in leisure activities.

_____ Getting involved in illegal activities or criminal behaviors.

_____ Other self-defeating behaviors (write in your own examples).

_____

_____

The first step in changing self-destructive or self-defeating behaviors is to identify what they are. The previous examples should help you begin to identify which behaviors you may need to change. The next step is figuring out a specific plan of action to help you change one or more of your patterns of behavior. Use the following examples to guide you in beginning to look at how you can change one behavior.

Example #1: Shauntey's Self-defeating Relationship Pattern

I have a long pattern of getting hooked up with men who take advantage of me. They use me for sex and to get money and drugs from me. A couple guys have even beat me up, but I stuck with them because I didn't want to be alone and thought I could change them.

I'm working on changing this relationship pattern. The first thing I have to do is go slow in developing any new relationships with men. I can no longer let myself get sexually and emotionally involved with men who I hardly know because I always end up getting used and hurt. Also, there's no way I can get involved with a man who gets high because I'm too vulnerable and likely to let him drag me down. I'll work on developing friendships first. Then if any other type of relationship follows, I'll be in better shape emotionally to handle it.

Example #2: Rob's Self-destructive Pattern of Aggressiveness

For years I've been getting into fights with other dudes. I can't tell you how many people I messed up or how many times I've been whipped real bad. My pattern has been to retaliate and "get even" with anyone who does me wrong. I never even cared if I got hurt. Hell, I not only been beat up real bad, but I even got stabbed twice. It didn't use to matter to me 'cause I ain't never been scared of no one. But I'm getting too old for this. I'm tired of the streets and fighting all the time.

There's a couple things I can do to change. First thing is to stay off all chemicals, especially crack, 'cause that stuff makes me even more aggressive than I usually am. But booze messes with me real bad, too, so I got to stay off it, as well. I gotta change my nasty attitude. I can cop a bad attitude in a minute, and I know this only gets me fired up and ready to fight. I also gotta stop gettin' in peoples' faces when I disagree with them. I been in jail a couple times and the forensic unit of a mental hospital once and I had enough. I got two kids who are doing real good, and I want to see them get to college 'cause I ain't never even finished high school. If I still live with the street mentality I just ain't gonna make it. It's just a matter of time. A real key is going to therapy and NA meetings and sticking with them, 'cause in the past I always stop when I hear the truth from a therapist or sponsor about my attitude and nastiness.

Behavior Change

One example of a behavior from the previous list I want to change is:

_____

_____

Steps I can take to change this behavior are:

_____

_____

_____

_____

Benefits of making this change are:

_____

_____

_____

_____

SESSION 23
Changing Personality Traits

Changing personality traits is an excellent way of self-improvement. In the 12-Step programs, much attention is directed to changing "defects of character," which refers to the need to make changes in your personality as a way of helping your recovery and making you a better person. Many people with psychiatric disorders and addiction have a personality disorder, which refers to having a group of personality traits that cause difficulty in life or considerable personal distress. However, even if you don't have a personality disorder, you too can benefit from improving your personality.

Personality traits refer to the way you view and relate to the world. These traits show in your attitudes and behaviors and play a major role in your ability to function in life and get along with other people. Because your traits are "ingrained," they will take time to change. Remember, you can always work on changing traits that get you into difficulty with others as well as develop positive aspects of your personality. But like other changes, it takes time, effort, a willingness to work at self-improvement, and a plan of action to guide you in the change process.

Some personality traits can be seen in terms of "opposites." For each trait there often is another trait that is somewhat of an opposite one. For example, the opposite of "self-centered" is being "other-centered," the opposite of "patient" is "impatient," and the opposite of "perfectionistic" is being "chaotic or scattered." It isn't whether or not you have a particular trait but the degree to which you have the trait and how it affects your sense of self and your relationships with others that determines if it is a problem for you.

This brief list of traits may or may not describe you most of the time. Place a ✓ next to any trait that you think causes serious problems for you.

_____ *Passive* — letting things happen to me without speaking my mind, letting others take advantage of me, and holding my thoughts and feelings inside.

_____ *Aggressive* — letting my thoughts and feelings out without regard for others, being pushy with others, or being verbally or physically intrusive.

_____ *Shy and inhibited* — it's hard to talk or share things with others or let others get close to me.

_____ *Uninhibited* — saying or doing whatever I want without thinking about the impact of my actions on others.

123

_____ *Self-centered* — seeing things mainly from my point of view and not focusing on other people's ideas, feelings, or needs.

_____ *Other-centered* — focusing too much time and energy on taking care of others and meeting their needs, often at the expense of ignoring my own needs.

_____ *Impulsive* — acting before I think about the consequences of my behavior, doing what I want when I want to, and doing whatever suits me at the moment.

_____ *Controlling* — wanting to be in control of situations and people and do things my way and having trouble letting others make decisions or give input.

_____ *Perfectionistic* — wanting things to be "just right," having high expectations, or having difficulty making mistakes or failing at anything or coping with things that don't meet my high standards.

_____ *Antisocial* — conning, taking advantage of or manipulating other people to get what I want from them, breaking the rules and laws as I see fit, or not caring about hurting other people.

_____ *Conscientious* — being concerned about what I do and my impact on other people, wanting to do the right thing or do a good job at whatever I am involved in.

_____ *Dependent* — difficulty making decisions on my own and depending too much on others for my sense of self, or having trouble doing things without the constant need for others to guide me.

_____ *Independent* — able to make decisions on my own, solve problems, and get my needs satisfied without leaning too much on others.

_____ *Cold or aloof* — being detached emotionally from other people, having trouble getting close or sharing positive feelings, or having problems caring for others.

_____ *Kind or caring* — giving of myself to others, really caring about what other people do or feel, sharing my time, energy, or resources with others.

_____ *Impatient* — having difficulty waiting, wanting things to be done right away, having trouble delaying my needs or gratification, or becoming annoyed with others who move too slowly or who don't do things the way I think they should.

_____ *Patient* — able to wait or delay getting my needs satisfied.

_____ *Irresponsible* — not taking care of my responsibilities or obligations, not being dependable with others, or doing whatever I want to do.

_____ *Overly responsible* — spending too much time and energy making sure things get done and other people get taken care of, worrying too much about things being right, or taking on too many responsibilities.

_____ *Suspicious or jealous* — being guarded around others, not trusting their motives, or always keeping others under my watchful eye for fear they may do something that I don't like.

_____ *Insensitive* — not being able to care about or be concerned about the needs and feelings of others, or not caring how I affect them with what I say or do.

_____ *Sensitive* — caring about the needs and feelings of others, or trying to understand things from their point of view.

_____ *Persistent* — able to stick with things even when the going gets rough.

This is just a partial list of some personality traits and examples of the behavior patterns in which these traits show. There are many other traits as well.

1.   In the space below, write in other personality traits that you think you want to work on changing or developing.

_____

_____

_____

_____

_____

2.   Choose one trait from the items that you checked or from your answers to question #1 that you want to begin working on changing or developing. Write this trait below and list a few steps that you can take to help you change this trait:

One personality trait I want to change is:

_____

Steps I can take to change this trait are:

_____

_____

_____

_____

Maria's Need to Control Others

I'm definitely too controlling and always want things to be my way. I badger my husband all the time to do things that I think he should do. I even try to tell him how to dress. This is going to be real hard to change. But I can start by cutting down on all the lists I give my husband of things to do around the house. It's like I'm always keeping him busy doing things at home. I can also let him and the children choose recreational activities they like instead of me being the one who always makes the decision. I can change this by not making critical remarks about what my husband is wearing when we go out because all this is is another way to control him and get him to wear what I think he should wear.

Jackson's Tendency to Be
Too Nice and Tolerant of Others

I'm too nice and tolerant of other people and end up getting taken advantage of as a result. I have to learn how to say no sometimes when other people ask me to do things that I don't want to do. I also have to express my opinion and feelings when people do things that irk me. Like with my brother — he's always late when we decide to go somewhere together and he often borrows money, seldom paying it back on time like he promises. I'm too nice with my kids, too, and let them take advantage of me by getting extra money for me or getting out of doing chores they are supposed to do. I'm going to have to put my foot down because I let resentments build up inside when I let my family or friends take advantage of me. It's not that I want to become hard-nosed all the time, it's just that I have to quit being so damn nice all the time.

SESSION 24
Changing My Thinking

The way you think affects your mood. The "internal messages" you give yourself can contribute to feeling anxious, bored, depressed, or miserable. Or these messages can lead to feeling happy, confident, and satisfied.

How you think also affects how you act. You can talk yourself into acting in certain ways. For example, you can talk yourself into working hard at your job and succeed as a result of using your self-talk to motivate yourself. Or you can give yourself messages that you are incompetent and talk yourself into messing up on the job.

Negative thinking can also contribute to relapse to alcohol or other drug use. It can be a factor in relapse to psychiatric illness, too.

On the other hand, positive thinking helps you to feel better and improve your relationships and your life. Thinking more positively can help you solve problems, feel more confident about your abilities, and feel more hopeful about your life. Learning to increase positive thinking can greatly aid your recovery.

Learning to identify and change your negative thinking is a helpful recovery strategy. Changing your negative thinking can lead to positive changes in your moods and behaviors.

Following are examples of negative thinking associated with addiction, psychiatric illness, or dual disorders. Place a ✓ next to the statements that you think more often than not represent typical ways you think about yourself and your life.

_____ I usually make things out worse than they really are or make "mountains out of molehills."

_____ I usually expect the worst possible thing to happen to me.

_____ I often expect to fail at the things I do.

_____ I tend to have many more negative than positive thoughts.

_____ I tend to have too many negative thoughts about myself or my abilities.

_____ I usually focus on the negative side of a situation.

_____ I have trouble seeing the positive side of life.

_____ I don't think I have any positive qualities or much to offer others.

127

____ If people knew the real me, they wouldn't like me.

____ I don't think other people like me very much.

____ I often think I'm not capable of getting better.

____ I often think I'm not capable of making positive changes in my life.

____ I often think I'm not capable of staying off alcohol or other drugs.

____ I keep bothersome thoughts to myself and don't let others know what I'm thinking.

____ I often think I need treatment for only a short period of time.

____ I dwell too much on my shortcomings or problems.

____ I worry too much about the future.

____ I often think that life isn't worth living.

____ I often think that a few drinks, joints, pills, lines, or hits off the crack pipe couldn't really hurt me.

____ I think I'll hurt someone if I don't learn to control my angry or violent thoughts.

Recovery Activity

Choose two statements from this list and write these in the spaces below. Then, for each one, list two new, positive thoughts.

Negative Thought #1: _____

_____

Two New, Positive Thoughts:
(1) _____
(2) _____

Negative Thought #2: _____

_____

Two New, Positive Thoughts:
(1) _____
(2) _____

Countering Negative Thoughts

Changing negative thoughts takes time and practice just like all of the other recovery tasks. Here are some suggested strategies that may help you decrease your negative thinking and increase your positive thinking.

- *Be aware of your negative thought patterns.*

  Catch yourself when you are thinking negatively. Becoming aware of your thoughts puts you in a position to challenge and change them.

- *Check the evidence for your negative thoughts.*

  When you make a statement such as "I'm not capable of change," make sure you closely check to see what evidence you have that this statement is true. Often you will find that it is not true in all situations. Even if it has been difficult for you to change, this doesn't mean you *can't* change. Or suppose you say to yourself, "I'm a failure at everything." If you closely check all the evidence, what you would find is that like everyone else you have made mistakes and had failures, but you have also succeeded at things. Remember, negative thinking tends to distort the "big picture," so checking out the facts and the evidence helps you to make a "reality check."

- *Challenge negative thinking.*

  When you are having negative thoughts, challenge them. For example, if you have a job interview coming up and think, "I'm going to do poorly and lose this job possibility," tell yourself instead, "If I prepare for the job interview, I'll feel more confident." Or suppose you are going to visit your parents and think, "I'm going to have a rotten time." Challenge this by saying, "It doesn't always go well when I visit Mom and Dad, but I'm going to make the best of it. Besides, even though they complain a lot, I know deep down they like my company and really need to see me."

- *Practice positive thinking over and over every day.*

  Each day try to increase the number of positive thoughts you have, no matter how small they seem. Make it a point to give yourself positive messages such as "I'm going to have a good day," "I'm going to enjoy myself," "I can cope with my problems," or "I have problems, but I have a lot of things going well for me, too." Even if you have to force yourself to say nice or positive things each day, make it a point to do so.

- *Focus less on the negative and more on the positive side of a situation.*

Instead of always seeing the glass as "half empty" and seeing the negative side of things, look at the other side. Remind yourself of the positive. For example, suppose your AA/NA sponsor or a family member gave you some critical feedback about how you were setting yourself up to relapse. Instead of having negative thoughts about them and yourself, you might say instead, "It's hard to hear the truth, but they were right in what they said to me. Just because they criticized me doesn't mean I'm not capable of doing OK or that I'm a bad person. It also doesn't mean they are jerks because they told me something that was hard to hear."

- *Allow room for mistakes.*

Don't expect perfection from yourself or not to make mistakes. Learn from your mistakes instead of using them to make yourself feel guilty or incompetent. It is very common to make mistakes when trying new behaviors or skills. Learning to think more positively and less negatively is no exception, so give yourself room to make errors.

- *Review your progress and accomplishments.*

Sometimes you can counter negative thoughts by reviewing your progress and accomplishments. When you are having a rough time, this can help you see the "bigger picture." Even if things don't always go well, that doesn't mean you don't deserve to compliment yourself for the efforts you put forth in recovery. Look for even small steps toward change, and don't expect major changes to happen overnight. Taking a daily or weekly inventory can help you regularly review your progress.

- *Remind yourself of the benefits of recovery.*

There are many benefits to recovery, even if it may not seem this way at a given time. Reminding yourself of the actual or potential benefits of recovery can help you during times you think things are going too slow or things aren't going well. This can help you see the "big picture" and the long-term benefits of recovery from dual disorders.

- *Make positive statements to others.*

One way to decrease negative and increase positive thinking is to say positive things about others or directly to them. For example, let's say your children came home with report cards that weren't as good as you had hoped. Rather than get critical, you might compliment them for their good grades and tell them you want to help them work at bringing up some of their other grades. Or suppose a friend or co-worker does something nice for you. Tell them you appreciate what they did.

130

- *Write in a journal.*

  Keep a written journal in which you write down positive thoughts or positive things that happen to you. Try to write at least a couple of positive statements each day, no matter how small they seem to be.

- *Continue to read recovery literature.*

  Many good books exist related to recovery and dual disorders that can help you continue to learn ways to make positive changes in your thinking. Books by Dr. David Burns, Dr. Aaron Beck, and Dr. Albert Ellis are especially helpful. Check Appendix 1 at the end of this workbook. Go to your local library or a bookstore. Or ask your therapist or doctor for other readings.

- *Recite the slogans or the Serenity Prayer.*

  Slogans used in AA/NA such as "This too will pass," "Think before you drink [or drug]," or "One day at a time" can help you get through rough times.

SESSION 25
Developing My Spirituality

An important aspect of recovery involves your spirituality. Defined broadly, spirituality refers to your "higher self." It involves your values and the relationships and activities in your life that bring you meaning, purpose, and direction. Spirituality also involves your beliefs about God or a Higher Power and your religious practices. Although you do not have to be associated with a "formal" religion to be spiritual, many people do find it helpful to participate in a specific religion. Attending services and other religious practices bring much comfort to many people.

For some people, being of service to others is a major way of showing their spiritual nature. This may show in the work they do for a living or helping others by serving as a volunteer in some community program or organization (for example, at a nursing home, hospital, addiction treatment program, prison, as a "big brother" or "big sister," etc.). In 12-Step recovery programs, people serve others by becoming a "sponsor." There are many ways you can be of service to others.

An important aspect of spirituality is that recovery is a *we process* more than an *I process*. Therefore, becoming connected with and relying on other people and God (or a Higher Power) can greatly aid your ongoing recovery. By sharing your recovery with others and working a "we" program, you not only *get* hope, strength, and support from others, you *give* it to others as well.

Here are some questions to help you focus on developing your spirituality:

1.   What relationships, activities, or values give you the most meaning and purpose in your life at this time? Explain your answer below.

_____

_____

_____

_____

_____

_____

_____

_____

2. Describe your own view of spirituality and what this means to you in recovery:

_____
_____
_____
_____
_____
_____

3. Describe ways you are currently—or would like to be—of service to other people:

_____
_____
_____
_____
_____
_____

4. Identify one area related to your spirituality that you would like to change or develop. Then, state some steps you can take to work toward these changes:

_____
_____
_____
_____
_____
_____

Some Ways to Develop Your Spirituality

- Rely on God or your Higher Power for strength, guidance, purpose in life, and understanding.

- Participate in religious services and other religious activities.

- Make praying a regular part of your day or join a prayer group.

- Attend a religious retreat or spend time at a monastery or other spiritual place to get in touch with yourself and your spiritual beliefs.

- Meditate.

- Read the Bible or other spiritual and inspirational guides to seek knowledge, guidance, and motivation.

- Discuss spirituality issues in therapy sessions or with your AA/NA sponsor.

- Focus on the 12-Step program, especially Steps 2, 3, 4, 5, 6, 7, 11, and 12.

- Seek spiritual advice from a priest, minister, rabbi, or other religious person.

- Focus on the greater good of society and contributions that you can make to make the world a better place.

- Be of service to others.

- Show love and compassion in your daily life in your interactions with other people.

- Be kind and forgiving to people you believe have hurt you.

- Accept your own weaknesses and limitations, and be kind to yourself and tolerant of your shortcomings and mistakes.

- If you feel guilty for things you've done that have hurt others, stop the hurtful behavior and decide if you need to make amends to undo some of the damage.

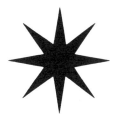

SECTION VII

Making
Lifestyle Changes

SESSION 26
My Daily Plan for Recovery

A daily plan includes the steps you are taking to abstain from using alcohol or drugs and cope with your psychiatric problem. It includes the "tools of recovery" you will use and how you will spend your time.

Place a √ next to the following recovery tools you use at least on a weekly basis:

____ AA, NA, CA meetings or other addiction support group meetings

____ Mental health and dual recovery support group meetings

____ Discussions with a sponsor (phone or face-to-face)

____ Working the 12-Step program of AA/NA/DRA

____ Discussions with other people in recovery

____ Individual or group therapy sessions

____ Sessions with my psychiatrist

____ Taking medications for a psychiatric problem

____ Praying or using a Higher Power

____ Reading recovery literature

____ Writing in a journal or recovery workbook

____ Talking myself through cravings or desires to get high

____ Practicing positive thinking

____ Having fun in alcohol- and drug-free environments

____ Other recovery tools (write in): _____

_____

_____

List three benefits of regularly using your recovery tools:

(1) _____

(2) _____

(3) _____

List possible negative consequences of not using your recovery tools regularly:

(1) _____

(2) _____

(3) _____

In early recovery, many people find it helpful to structure their days and their weeks. This helps to build recovery activities and fun into your week. The more active you are, and the less bored you are, the better your chances of staying alcohol or drug free.

If you don't regularly get involved in recovery activities or use the recovery tools listed on the previous page, you increase the chances of a relapse. You can use the blank **Daily Schedule** on the next page to help you begin structuring your week.

My Daily Schedule

	Sunday	Monday	Tuesday	Wednesday	Thursday	Friday	Saturday
6:00							
7:00							
8:00							
9:00							
10:00							
11:00							
12:00							
1:00							
2:00							
3:00							
4:00							
5:00							
6:00							
7:00							
8:00							
9:00							
10:00							
11:00							

SESSION 27
Setting Goals

Setting goals to work toward is an important part of life. Having goals can give you direction in life and help focus your time and energy. Working hard at reaching your goals, even if you don't reach them all, gives you a sense of satisfaction and accomplishment. It can make you feel better about yourself, too. On the other hand, without any goals in life you are more likely to feel useless, bored, or depressed. And your life is more likely to lack direction and structure which can raise the risk of relapse to alcohol or other drug use.

A goal refers to a process, a purpose, or some end that you wish to achieve. A goal can relate to learning information, increasing your skills, or changing something about yourself, your relationships, or your lifestyle.

Goals can be general or specific. For example, a **general goal** could be to "become a better parent." A **specific goal** would be to "get closer to my son by teaching him how to play a sport." Another example of a general goal is to "become a better worker." A more specific goal would be to "learn how to use a computer so I am more efficient at my job." "Losing weight and getting in shape" would be another general goal, whereas "losing fifteen pounds by the beginning of summer" would be a more specific goal.

Goals can be short, medium, or long term. A short-term goal is something you want to achieve within three months, a medium-term goal is something you want to achieve in three to six months, and a long-term goal is something you want to achieve in six months or longer. Some goals are a one-shot deal, such as saving a specific amount of money, going on a specific vacation, completing a particular project, or finishing a training program. Other goals are ongoing, especially goals related to changing yourself. For example, becoming more kind and loving or becoming a better spouse or parent is an ongoing goal that you continuously work at. Usually it is good to have a variety of goals that you are working toward. However, try to avoid setting too many goals or setting ones that are unreachable, because if you do this you will set yourself up to feel bad if you don't achieve them.

Goals not only give you structure and a sense of purpose or direction, but they can become a yardstick to measure your progress against. For example, suppose you are lonely and isolated and set a goal of developing two new friendships within the next several months. If you actually develop these relationships, you will know that you reached your goal.

Once you state your general or specific goal, then you need to figure out steps you can take to reach your goal. These steps become your **plan of action**. Let's say, for example, that you set a general goal of "becoming closer to your family." You then have to figure out how to go about getting closer to your family. Perhaps you may accomplish this goal by regularly visiting family members, inviting them to visit you, calling them on the phone, writing letters to them, sharing social activities together, or taking an interest in their lives.

Or let's say you set a goal of "getting along better with my daughter." You may accomplish this by spending more time with her, taking an interest in her day-to-day activities, helping her with her homework or special projects, taking her to a movie or some other fun activity, and telling her that you love her or care about her. You may also work toward this goal by eliminating or reducing behaviors that interfere with your relationship, such as snapping out angrily at her whenever she makes a mistake or belittling her if she doesn't do as well as you think she should in her schoolwork.

You can develop goals in virtually any area of your life. These areas, with a few examples, including the following:

- *Your addiction* — learning how to stay off drugs or cope with desires to get high.

- *Your psychiatric disorder* — learning how to cope with depression or negative thoughts about yourself.

- *Your family* — getting closer to your parents or becoming more actively involved in their lives.

- *Your marriage* — improving your ability to resolve differences and conflicts with your spouse or becoming more affectionate with your spouse.

- *Your friendships and relationships* — expanding your social network or making new friends with whom you can share interests.

- *Your interpersonal style* — learning to say no to others when you don't want to do things they ask of you or learning to express your ideas without worrying too much about what other people think.

- *Your physical health* — improving your diet, losing weight, or getting in better physical shape.

- *Your emotional health* — learning to express your angry feelings instead of stuffing them or learning how to express loving feelings toward others.

- *Your thinking* — learning to change negative thoughts or increase the number of positive thoughts you have each day.

- *Your personality* — becoming more patient, more outgoing, less impulsive, or less self-centered.

- *Your spirituality* — developing a relationship with God or your Higher Power or becoming more active in religion.

- *Your leisure time* — learning a new hobby or sport or spending more time having fun.

140

- *Your education or job* — working toward a degree or finishing a training program, or improving your job skills.

- *Your lifestyle* — spending more time relaxing and having fun and less time working or building structure in your daily life so you don't have too much free time without anything to do.

- *Your money* — learning how to budget your money, save for the future, or save a specific amount of money for a specific reason such as to take a trip or purchase something that you want.

After setting goals and developing an initial plan of action, it is a good idea to run some of your ideas past your therapist, sponsor, or a friend. This gives you a chance to get their input and feedback about your goals and your plan. It is also helpful to review your goals so you can measure your progress. If you aren't making much progress, then try to figure out if your goal is too high or unrealistic. Also, try to figure out if your plan needs to be changed or if there are other barriers to reaching your goals. It isn't unusual for goals and steps to be modified as time goes on.

Be sure to reward yourself—both for progress toward reaching your goals and for efforts you put forth. Even if you don't reach a particular goal, if you've done your best, then be happy with your efforts. Some goals are going to be harder to reach than others. Don't be afraid of failure, either. *You can't grow as a person if you don't make mistakes.*

Overview of Setting Goals

- Set goals in your life so you have things you are working toward.

- Define your goals as specifically as you can.

- Once you set a goal, make a plan of steps you can take to reach it.

- Share your plan with others to get feedback from them or additional ideas on steps to take to reach your goals.

- If you aren't reaching your goals, try to figure out whether they are too unrealistic, your plan needs to be changed, or if you aren't working hard enough to reach your goals.

- Evaluate your progress from time to time so that you can change your goals or plans as needed.

- Give yourself credit for reaching your goals or for putting forth effort at working toward reaching goals, even if you don't always reach them.

Setting Goals

1. One **short-term goal** I want to achieve within the next three months is:

   _____

   _____

   Steps I can take to reach this goal include:

   _____

   _____

   _____

   _____

2. One **medium-term goal** I want to achieve within the next three to six months is:

   _____

   _____

   Steps I can take to reach this goal include:

   _____

   _____

   _____

   _____

3. One **long-term goal** I want to achieve within the next six to twelve months is:

   _____

   _____

   Steps I can take to reach this goal include:

   _____

   _____

   _____

SESSION 28
Financial Recovery

One of the areas often ignored during recovery is one's money or finances. Very frequently, addiction causes financial problems as a result of money spent for alcohol or other drugs. Those with an addiction to expensive drugs or gambling, for example, often pile up heavy debts. Financial problems are also caused by missing work or losing a job. It is not uncommon for alcoholics or drug addicts to be behind in paying their bills or even broke. Some even end up losing everything they ever owned.

Your family also may have experienced serious financial difficulties because of your addiction, particularly if you were the main source of income. Because of the financial drain of addiction, some families even have trouble meeting their basic needs for medical or dental care, housing, food, clothing, education, and recreation. These financial problems also can affect your family's mental well-being and self-esteem. A lack of consistent income, low income, or poor money management can lead to anxiety and feelings of insecurity with your family.

Answer the following questions to help you plan for your financial recovery:

1. How much money would you estimate you spent on alcohol or other drugs during the:

    past month? _____

    past year? _____

    entire course of your addiction? _____

2. How much income would you estimate you lost due to missing work or losing jobs as a result of your addiction? _____

3. How much of a drug debt, or court/lawyer expenses do you still have?

    _____

4. Describe other ways you and your family were affected financially by your addiction.

    _____

    _____

    _____

5. Describe what steps you can take to begin getting your financial situation in order.

    _____

    _____

    _____

Financial issues can be discussed with your counselor or AA/NA/DRA sponsor. Don't hesitate to seek the advice of a financial counselor if you think your situation warrants this. You may even wish to learn how to budget your money or manage a checking and/or savings account. (Session 29 will give you detailed information on handling money and debts.)

Some addicts associate having money with getting high. They feel they are more at risk to use if they have enough money for drugs. This attitude reflects **denial** and **stinking thinking**. If you think like this, be sure to talk about it with your counselor and/or sponsor.

Setting a Goal

My *Goal* in relation to my financial recovery is:

_____

_____

Steps I will take to reach this goal are:

_____

_____

_____

Potential benefits of reaching my goal are:

_____

_____

_____

SESSION 29
Strategies for Handling Money and Debt

- *Keep track of your spending.*

    In order to get a handle on where your money goes, keep track of all your spending for a couple months. This will help you more clearly see spending patterns. Perhaps you are spending a lot more on certain things than you thought.

    For example, in tracking your spending you might discover that you spend $70 more per month for food than you thought you were spending. Or you might find out that you are spending far too much money on clothes. Tracking your spending can help you figure out areas where you can cut down. Using a budget book is an excellent way of tracking your spending and keeping a running account of how you spend your money.

- *Develop and follow a budget.*

    A budget helps you to see the "big picture" in terms of how your income is used. Knowing where your money goes can help you figure out how you might need to cut back on spending. Keeping a budget also is a great way of being able to check your progress toward financial goals such as saving money or reducing debts.

    Following a budget can help you prepare for expenses such as car insurance or holiday gifts. Review your budget at least monthly to help you see where your money is going and to help you identify changes in spending habits that are needed.

    If you are on a limited income or live on public assistance or SSI, it is especially important to have a budget in order to make your limited income stretch.

- *Live within your financial means.*

    If you are spending more money than you are making or bringing in, then you are not living within your means. The longer you continue spending more money than you bring in, the deeper in debt you will go. Following a budget and developing a long-term financial plan are two ways of helping you figure out ways to live within your means.

- *Review your progress regularly.*

    It is a good idea to review your financial plan every week. This will help you determine if you are reaching your goals or if you need to change your goals or methods in reaching them. If your financial situation changes substantially, your plan will probably have to be modified to take into account the nature of this new change.

- *Eliminate or reduce loans and charge cards.*

Much money is wasted in interest paid on loans and charge cards. Charge cards in particular usually have very high interest rates that vary from 12 percent to more than 20 percent. Loans may also have high interest rates. There are certain financial lenders whose interest rates are just as high or even higher than credit card interest rates.

Paying off loans and credit cards is one of the first steps to getting your financial house in order. Not only does this prevent money from being wasted in paying interest charges, but this also reduces the amount of money you have to pay out of your budget every month to meet the loan or credit card payments.

You can take a "preventative" approach in relation to loans and credit cards. While loans and credit card purchases are sometimes necessary, there are many cases where they are not. If you are buying something with a credit card, for example, ask yourself if you would buy that item if you had the cash—do you *really* need it? Guard against impulsive buying with credit cards.

- *Avoid high interest loans or loan sharks.*

If you borrow from a loan shark, you will pay extremely high interest, and this will only throw you deeper in debt. If at all possible, avoid borrowing from places that charge high rates of interest (12 percent or more) because you will pay a lot back in interest charges.

- *Shop around for the best interest rates if you need a loan.*

If you need a loan for a car, home improvement, or for some other reason, check with different lending institutions to find out their interest rates. They often vary as much as a couple percent. A difference of 1 percent on a car loan, for example, can mean saving $10–20 a month on your car payment. This may not seem like much of a savings, but if you multiply the number of months you make car payments, your savings can add up.

- *Avoid aimless shopping and impulsive buying.*

An easy way to get in debt and accumulate bills is going shopping when you don't need something in particular and you simply wish to "look around." If you avoid aimless shopping, you substantially decrease the chances of impulsive buying or buying something on the spur of the moment because it has attracted your interest or attention. Most things bought on impulse are not things you *need* but things you *want* or *think you need*.

- *Think ahead to the future.*

It is a good idea to think ahead to the future and regularly put aside money, even if this is only a small amount. The years fly by more quickly than you realize. Thinking ahead helps you plan for your future, whether it relates to buying a house or car, financing your child's education, or planning for your retirement.

Most employers offer retirement programs. If your employer's retirement program allows you to have contributions withheld from your paycheck, make sure you do this rather than take the money in your paycheck. This not only helps build for your future financial security but probably also helps to reduce your current tax liability as well. There are many people who regret not contributing to a retirement fund offered by their company.

To protect your family, it is also good to have life insurance and disability insurance. If you are the sole support of your family, their security could be greatly jeopardized if you got a serious injury or illness and couldn't work, or if you died.

- *Figure out ways to cut down expenses and increase savings.*

There are a lot of little ways you can cut down your expenses and increase the money available for debt reduction or saving. Here are just a few examples:

- Buy food items and other household items in bulk quantity. Look for special sales or discount stores. You often can save anywhere from 30–50 percent or even more by buying in bulk or by buying a large size of a product. If you are on a limited income and cannot afford to buy in large quantities, get some friends to pitch in together to buy bulk quantities so that you all can stretch your money.

- Buy generic food and medicine products. This can also save you a substantial amount of money. For example, a name brand aspirin product may cost you $7 and the exact same generic product may cost you less than $4.

- Look for things you need at yard sales, garage sales, estate sales, or advertised for sale by individuals in the newspaper. For example, a new bicycle for your child may cost anywhere from $80–150. You may find a bicycle in good shape at a yard sale or in a newspaper ad for less than $25.

- A few other easy ways to reduce expenses include: taking your lunch to work, car pooling to work, using the library instead of buying books, shopping from a list and buying only items on your list, not shopping on an empty stomach, and renting items you seldom use instead of buying them. For example, rather than buy a videotape for $20 or more, rent it for a buck or so whenever you feel like watching it.

- *Use a financial counselor or consultant if needed.*

If you are over your head in debt or overwhelmed with financial matters, it can help to discuss your situation with a financial counselor or consultant. This individual can help you figure out your financial plan, whether it's simply to get control over your debts or to develop an investment plan for the future.

- *Develop a financial plan (short and long term).*

Money is no different from any other area of life: if you develop goals and specific plans to reach them, you are more likely to achieve them. A plan gives you a sense of direction. Your plan should be in writing and include short- and long-term goals.

If you are married or involved in a close relationship in which money and assets are shared, this plan should be developed jointly with your spouse or partner so that you both have input and agree on strategies. Working together is essential if a plan is to be developed in a way that considers both of your ideas and interests. It also gives you a greater chance that your plan will actually be followed.

SECTION VIII

Maintaining Gains
and
Preventing Relapse

The Importance of Follow-up After
Rehabilitation or Hospital-based Treatment

Before your rehabilitation or hospital stay is completed you will work with your treatment team to develop a follow-up plan. This plan addresses the problems and issues you need to continue working on once you leave residential or hospital care. It outlines the specific things you need to change and your involvement in other community programs or services. Your family or other important people in your life may also be asked to participate in developing this plan.

Your ongoing plan may involve continued care in another inpatient or residential facility, a day hospital program, outpatient services, self-help programs, and the use of medications. All of these are discussed in sections that follow.

Other Inpatient Programs

Your treatment team may recommend further inpatient care following your current hospital stay. Examples of these inpatient programs include state hospitals, halfway houses, rehabilitation programs, or community living programs. The amount of time spent in these programs depends on your illnesses and your personal goals.

Partial Programs (Day Hospital)

Some patients who leave the hospital or a residential rehabilitation program still require intensive involvement in treatment but do not need a residential program. Outpatient treatment is simply not enough for them. A "partial" hospital or "intensive outpatient" program where they participate in treatment for several hours a day, several days per week, may be recommended.

The purpose of partial hospital programs is to ease the transition between the hospital and independent living. Many of the same treatment services available in the hospital—group therapy, specialized treatment groups, and activities—are offered at partial programs. You may also participate in individual and family therapy sessions. The support provided by the staff and other patients often helps adapting to life outside of the hospital. Such support also makes it easier for you to work on personal problems.

These programs may be connected with a psychiatric treatment facility or a chemical dependency facility. Depending on the program you attend, the primary focus may be on your psychiatric disorder, your addiction, or both.

Outpatient Services

If your illness was severe enough to require an inpatient stay in a psychiatric or chemical dependency program, then follow-up outpatient care will be needed. Outpatient care helps you to continue building on the gains you made while in the hospital. It also helps you deal with the problems and adjustments you will face as you continue your recovery from dual disorders.

There are different types of outpatient treatment. These include individual, group, and family therapy. You may receive outpatient care from a private professional such as a psychiatrist, psychologist, or other mental health professional, a community-based mental health center, drug and alcohol clinic, or other type of agency.

For many people symptoms of psychiatric illness and/or addiction come back. Involvement in outpatient care helps you spot the warning signs early and help you to either prevent a relapse or get the help you need should a relapse occur. It is important to keep your outpatient appointments, even if you feel a lot better than before you went to the hospital. Stopping outpatient care too early can contribute to a relapse.

Medications

Many types of psychiatric illness require taking medications, even after the symptoms of your illness are under control. You need to see a psychiatrist on a regular basis if you are on medicine. A common relapse warning sign is stopping medications without first discussing this with your doctor or the others providing treatment. If you feel you no longer need or want to take medication, talk it over with your doctor or therapist.

For acute episodes of illness, it is often recommended that you stay on medication for at least four to six months after your symptoms go away. If you've experienced recurrent episodes of your illness or have a chronic form of psychiatric illness, it is recommended that you remain on your medicine as a way of reducing the future possibility of another episode.

Special medications are sometimes used in the treatment of addiction as well. Some alcoholics use a medication called disulfiram (Antabuse). This drug stays in the system up to 10–14 days after the last dose is taken. If an alcoholic drinks while on this medication, he or she will get very sick. The idea behind this is if Antabuse is in one's system and there is a desire to drink, drinking may be put off until the Antabuse is out of the system. This essentially buys the alcoholic time, and often within a few hours or days the desire to drink leaves.

Opiate addicts sometimes take a drug called naltrexone (Trexan), which blocks the euphoric affects of opiate drugs. The idea behind this is that if heroin or another opiate drug is used while taking naltrexone, the high won't be experienced. This in turn will discourage the addict from future episodes of opiate use. There are some drugs used to decrease the craving for cocaine use. These include medications called bromocriptine and amantadine. Any medication used for the treatment of addiction should be seen as an adjunct to therapy and counseling and self-help programs.

Self-Help Programs

Many people have found self-help programs to be very beneficial to their ongoing recovery. Most communities offer self-help programs for psychiatric illness as well as alcohol and drug problems. Self-help programs are groups of people with similar problems or illnesses helping each other out. They meet regularly to discuss their illnesses and problems, as well as steps they can take to overcome these. For example, many groups use a 12-Step recovery program, which is a suggested way of viewing your problems and recovery from them.

There are different types of self-help meetings. Some are **speaker meetings** in which a person talks about his or her illness and recovery. Others are **discussion meetings** in which common problems or concerns are discussed. You can go to as many meetings as you need. Some people, for example, go every day. Others go once or twice a week.

Self-help programs can provide you with a guide, often referred to as a **sponsor**. A sponsor is someone recovering from one or more illnesses who can "teach you the ropes" about the program. This is someone who will attend meetings with you, guide you through working the 12 Steps, or talk with you by telephone when you need a friendly voice.

You should get a list of programs available in your community before you leave the hospital or rehabilitation program. You may need to attend many meetings at different locations before you find one or more to attend on a regular basis.

Self-help meetings are also available for your family. You may wish to speak with them about attending meetings.

Rehospitalization

While many people never return to the hospital for treatment, some do when the symptoms of their psychiatric illness become severe or they get hooked again on alcohol or other drugs. Involvement in outpatient care makes it easier to go back for inpatient treatment should your symptoms require this. The reality is that some people will require future hospitalizations to manage acute episodes of their illness. The next session will discuss relapse in greater detail.

SESSION 31
Relapse Warning Signs

There are many warning signs of relapse to both addiction and psychiatric illness that you should learn about. These warning signs may show gradually over a period of days, weeks, or even longer. Or they can show up rather quickly. Being aware of relapse warning signs puts you in a position to take action to do something about them so that you don't use alcohol or drugs and you lessen your chances of a full-blown relapse of your psychiatric symptoms.

Relapse warning signs may show in changes in your attitude, mood, behavior, and daily habits. Sometimes, relapse warning signs show in existing symptoms worsening because some symptoms may not go away totally. For example, Leslie has learned she can live with a certain degree of anxiety. However, when her anxiety level raises significantly for a few days and she starts to avoid going out of her house, she knows this is a relapse warning sign.

Warning signs may be obvious. For example, John knows he's headed back to drug use when he blows off NA meetings and calls guys he used to party with. Linda knows she's likely to experience her mania again when she stops taking her Lithium on her own without even discussing her condition with her therapist or doctor.

Warning signs can also be "sneaky" and not appear to relate to your dual disorders. For example, before Anthony uses alcohol or drugs again, he begins to become dishonest in small ways by lying to friends or family. In time, his dishonesty shows in scamming and conning others. Soon he's back to using drugs again.

Although everyone has his or her own set of warning signs, there are some common ones that many other people with dual disorders have experienced before an episode of psychiatric illness or alcohol and drug use. Use the list that follows to learn about these warning signs and help you develop your plan for coping with these signs of relapse.

If you have been in treatment before for either or both of your disorders, try to figure out which of the following warning signs may have been present before a relapse by placing a (✓) next to the signs you experienced. If this is your first time in recovery, check the signs below that you think could represent relapse warning signs in the future.

Attitude and Thought Changes

____   Losing interest in your recovery plan
____   Thinking treatment or medications aren't needed anymore
____   Not caring about yourself or what happens to your life
____   Increase in negative thinking about the future or your treatment

153

_____ Racing and confusing thoughts

_____ Paranoid thoughts

_____ Thinking about suicide

_____ Thinking about hurting someone else

_____ Thinking you can use "some" alcohol or drugs and stay in control or that using will help you feel better

_____ Missing the action of partying, using alcohol and drugs, or being with a "fast crowd"

_____ Increase in obsessive thoughts

_____ Thinking about ways to take advantage of others or break the law

Mood or Emotional Changes: Feeling More

_____ Sad or depressed

_____ Energetic, excited, "keyed up," or on top of the world

_____ Anxious, nervous, or on edge

_____ Fearful and afraid

_____ Guilty and shameful

_____ Bored, restless, or "empty"

_____ Shifts in moods from depression to mania

_____ Lonely

_____ Angry and hurt

Behavior Changes

_____ Missing or stopping treatment sessions with your therapist or doctor

_____ Cutting down or stopping AA, NA, dual recovery, or mental health support group meetings

_____ Cutting down or stopping your medications without first discussing this with your therapist or doctor

_____ Cutting down or stopping regular contact with a sponsor or other members of support groups

_____ Withdrawing from other people and keeping to yourself

_____ Arguing more with others

_____ Cutting down or stopping hobbies or enjoyable activities

_____ Putting yourself in situations where there is pressure to use alcohol or drugs

_____ Talking much slower or faster than usual or in a way that is confusing to others

_____ Dressing in strange or bizarre ways

___ Acting in strange or bizarre ways

___ Hurting yourself

___ Hurting someone else

___ Getting involved in illegal activities again

Health Habits or Daily Routine Changes

___ Sleeping a lot more or less than usual, or trouble falling or staying asleep

___ Big change in energy level (much higher or lower than usual)

___ Big change in appetite or eating habits (increase or decrease)

___ Cutting down or stopping regular exercise

___ Change in personal hygiene habits

___ Big change in your regular routines for the day or week

If there are any other relapse warning signs you've experienced before, write these here:

_____

_____

Gerald's Warning Signs and Coping Strategies

My biggest warning sign is thinking that I don't need medications, treatment, or support groups once I've been feeling good for a couple of months. To cope with these thoughts in the future I will: (1) immediately talk over these thoughts with my doctor or therapist; (2) ask myself why I am wanting to stop treatment to figure out what's really going on; (3) tell myself that I'm not going to make any decision to drop out of treatment for at least another month to buy myself more time; (4) discuss this feeling at the next meeting of the manic depression support group that I attend; (5) remind myself of how I do so much better when I stay on my medications and in treatment even during periods when I am doing well. I have to remind myself that I have a chronic disease that can only be treated by staying on medication and in treatment.

Recovery Exercise

Review the list of warning signs that you checked. In the spaces below, write down five possible warning signs of relapse for both your psychiatric illness and your addiction. Keep in mind some of these warning signs may be similar in both of your disorders.

Psychiatric Warning Signs	Addiction Warning Signs
(1)	(1)
(2)	(2)
(3)	(3)
(4)	(4)
(5)	(5)

Choose one psychiatric illness and one addiction relapse warning sign and list some steps you can take to help you cope with these warning signs. First, review the example of Gerald on the previous page to see one example of how you can do this recovery task.

Psychiatric Warning Sign: _____

_____

Three Coping Strategies:

   (1) _____

   (2) _____

   (3) _____

Addiction Warning Sign: _____

_____

Three Coping Strategies:

   (1) _____

   (2) _____

   (3) _____

Recovery Exercise

Review the list of warning signs that you checked. In the spaces below, write down five possible warning signs of relapse for both your psychiatric illness and your addiction. Keep in mind some of these warning signs may be similar in both of your disorders.

Psychiatric Warning Signs	Addiction Warning Signs
(1)	(1)
(2)	(2)
(3)	(3)
(4)	(4)
(5)	(5)

Choose one psychiatric illness and one addiction relapse warning sign and list some steps you can take to help you cope with these warning signs. First, review the example of Gerald on the previous page to see one example of how you can do this recovery task.

Psychiatric Warning Sign: _____

_____

Three Coping Strategies:

   (1) _____

   (2) _____

   (3) _____

Addiction Warning Sign: _____

_____

Three Coping Strategies:

   (1) _____

   (2) _____

   (3) _____

Recovery Exercise

1. Steps I can take if I use *any* alcohol or drugs are:

   _____

   _____

   _____

2. Steps I can take if I get *physically or mentally hooked* again are:

   _____

   _____

   _____

3. Steps I can take if my *psychiatric symptoms* worsen or return include:

   _____

   _____

   _____

4. I would need to go *into the hospital* for help if I experienced these symptoms or behaviors:

   _____

   _____

   _____

5. My *family, sponsor, or members of my recovery network* can help me by taking the following steps if I experience an emergency:

   _____

   _____

   _____

   Discuss your plan with people in your recovery network while you are doing well. Ask for help from your therapist or doctor in developing this plan.

APPENDIX 1
Suggested Readings

Alcoholics Anonymous ("Big Book"). New York: AA World Services, Inc., 1976.

Agras, S. *Facing Fears, Phobias and Anxiety*. New York: Freeman, 1985.

Beebe, Philip J. *The Codependent Counselor: Guidelines for Self-assessment and Change*. Independence, Missouri: Herald House/Independence Press, 1990.

Bell, Tammy. *Preventing Adolescent Relapse: A Guide for Parents, Teachers, and Counselors*. Independence, Missouri: Herald House/Independence Press, 1990.

Bourne, E. *The Anxiety and Phobia Workbook*. Oakland, California: New Harbinger Publications, Inc., 1990.

Burns, D. *Feeling Good: The New Mood Therapy*. New York: William Morrow, 1980.

Burns, D. *The Feeling Good Workbook*. New York: William Morrow, 1990.

Club, G.A. *Coping with Panic*. Belmont, California: Brooks/Cole, 1990.

Daley, Dennis. *Relapse Prevention Workbook*. Holmes Beach, Florida: Learning Publications, 1986.

Daley, D. *Surviving Addiction Workbook*. Holmes Beach, Florida: Learning Publications, 1990.

Daley, D. *Kicking Addictive Habits Once and For All: A Relapse Prevention Guide*. Lexington, Massachusetts: Lexington Press, 1991.

Daley, D. *Working Through Denial: The Key to Recovery*. Minneapolis, Minnesota: Johnson Institute, 1991.

Daley, D. *Coping with Anger Workbook*. Skokie, Illinois: Gerald T. Rogers Productions, 1992.

Daley, D. *Preventing Relapse*. Center City, Minnesota: Hazelden, 1993.

Daley, D. *Coping with Feelings Workbook*. Holmes Beach, Florida: Learning Publications, 1994.

Daley, D., and F. Campbell. *Coping with Dual Disorders* (2nd ed.). Center City, Minnesota: Hazelden, 1993.

Daley, D., and J. Sinberg. *A Family Guide to Dual Disorders* (2nd ed.). Center City, Minnesota: Hazelden, 1994.

Ellis, A. *How to Stubbornly Refuse to Make Yourself Miserable About Anything.* Secaucus, New Jersey: Lyle Stuart, 1988.

Glanz, L. *Overcoming Anxiety and Worry.* Skokie, Illinois: Gerald T. Rogers Productions, 1991.

Goodwin, D.W. *Anxiety.* New York: Oxford University Press, 1986.

Gorski, Terence T. *Getting Love Right: Learning the Choices of Healthy Intimacy.* Available from Herald House/Independence Press.

Gorski, T. *How to Start Relapse Prevention Support Groups.* Independence, Missouri: Herald House/Independence Press, 1989.

Gorski, T. *Keeping the Balance: A Psycho-spiritual Model of Personal Development.* Independence, Missouri: Herald House/Independence Press, 1993.

Gorski, T. *The Players and Their Personalities: Understanding People Who Get Involved in Addictive Relationships.* Independence, Missouri: Herald House/Independence Press, 1989.

Gorski, T. *The Staying Sober Workbook: A Serious Solution for the Problem of Relapse.* Independence, Missouri: Herald House/Independence Press, 1988.

Gorski, T. *Passages Through Recovery: An Action Plan for Preventing Relapse.* Center City, Minnesota: Hazelden, 1989.

Gorski, T. *Relapse Prevention Workbook for the Criminal Offender.* Independence, Missouri: Herald House/Independence Press, 1993.

Gorski, T. *The Relapse/Recovery Grid.* Independence, Missouri: Herald House/ Independence Press, 1989.

Gorski, T. *Understanding the Twelve Steps: A Guide for Counselors, Therapists, and Recovering People.* Independence, Missouri: Herald House/Independence Press, 1989.

Gorski, T., and Merlene Miller. *Staying Sober: A Guide for Relapse Prevention*. Independence, Missouri: Herald House/Independence Press, 1986.

Haskett, R.F., and D.C. Daley. *Understanding Manic Depressive Illness and Addiction*. Center City, Minnesota: Hazelden, 1994.

Howell, J., and M. Thase. *Beating the Blues: Recovery from Depression*. Skokie, Illinois: Gerald T. Rogers Productions, 1991.

Jeffers, S. *Feel the Fear and Do It Anyway*. New York: Fawcett Columbine, 1987.

Kelly, John M. *Out of the Fog: A Guide to Stabilization in Recovery*. Independence, Missouri: Herald House/Independence Press, 1992.

Kreisman, J., and H. Straus. *I Hate You—Don't Leave Me: Understanding the Borderline Personality*. New York: Avon Books, 1989.

Lerner, H. *The Dance of Anger*. New York: Harper and Row, 1985.

Lewinsohn, P., et al. *Control Your Depression*. New York: Prentice Hall, 1986.

Markway, B.G., et al. *Dying of Embarrassment: Help for Social Anxiety and Phobia*. Oakland, California: New Harbinger, 1992.

Martorano, J.T. *Beyond Negative Thinking: Breaking the Cycle of Depressing and Anxious Thoughts*. New York: Insight Books, 1989.

Miller, M., T. Gorski, and D. Miller. *Learning to Live Again: A Guide for Recovery from Chemical Dependency* (updated and revised ed.). Independence, Missouri: Herald House/Independence Press, 1992.

Narcotics Anonymous ("Basic Text"). Sun Valley, California: NA World Services, 1993.

Papolos, D., and J. Papolos. *Overcoming Depression*. New York: Harper and Row, 1987.

Rapoport, J.L. *The Boy Who Couldn't Stop Washing: The Experience and Treatment of Obsessive-Compulsive Disorder*. New York: New American Library, 1989.

Rosellini, G., and M. Worden. *Of Course You're Angry*. Center City, Minnesota: Hazelden, 1985.

Rosellini, G., and M. Worden. *Here Comes the Sun*. Center City, Minnesota: Hazelden, 1987.

Salloum, I., and D. Daley. *Understanding Anxiety Disorders and Addiction.* Center City, Minnesota: Hazelden, 1993.

Seagrave, A., and F. Covington. *Free From Fears: New Help for Anxiety, Panic and Agoraphobia.* New York: Poseidon Press, 1987.

Sheehan, D. *The Anxiety Disease.* New York: Charles Schribner and Sons, 1984.

Tauris, C. *Anger: The Misunderstood Emotion* (2nd ed.). New York: Simon and Schuster, 1989.

Thase, M., D. Daley. *Understanding Depression and Addiction.* Center City, Minnesota: Hazelden, 1993.

The Dual Recovery Book. Center City, Minnesota: Hazelden, 1993.

Trotter, Caryl. *Double Bind: A Guide to Recovery and Relapse Prevention for the Chemically Dependent Sexual Abuse Survivor.* Independence, Missouri: Herald House/Independence Press, 1992.

Weekes, C. *More Help for Your Nerves.* New York: Bantam Books, 1984.

Weiss, R., and D. Daley. *Understanding Personality Problems and Addiction.* Center City, Minnesota: Hazelden, 1994.

APPENDIX 2
Helpful Organizations

Alcoholics Anonymous World Services
Box 459, Grand Central Station
New York, NY 10163

Anxiety Disorders Association of America
6000 Executive Blvd., Suite 513
Rockville, MD 20852
(301) 231-9350

CHAANGE
128 County Club Drive
Chula Vista, CA 92011
(619) 425-3992

Depressive and Manic Depressive
  Association
222 South Riverside Plaza
Suite 2812
Chicago, IL 60606

Dual Recovery Anonymous
Central Service Office
P.O. Box 8107
Prairie Village, KS 66208

Emotional Health Anonymous
2420 San Gabriel Blvd.
Rosemead, CA 91770

GROW, Inc.
2403 West Springfield
Champaign, IL 61821

Narcotics Anonymous World Service Office
P.O. Box 9999
Van Nuys, CA 91409

National Alliance for the Mentally Ill
2101 Wilson Boulevard
Arlington, VA 22201

National Foundation for Depressive Illness
P.O. Box 2257
New York, NY 10116

Obsessive Compulsive Disorder Foundation,
  Inc.
P.O. Box 9573
New Haven, CT 06535

Phobic Society of America
P.O. Box 42514
Washington, DC 20015
(301) 231-9350

TERRAP Programs
648 Menlo Avenue, #5
Menlo Park, CA 94025
(415) 327-1312

Functional Anatomy for Sport and Exercise

A Quick A-to-Z Reference

Second Edition

Clare E. Milner

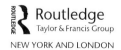

Routledge
Taylor & Francis Group

NEW YORK AND LONDON

Second edition published 2019
by Routledge
52 Vanderbilt Avenue, New York, NY 10017

and by Routledge
2 Park Square, Milton Park, Abingdon, Oxon, OX14 4RN

Routledge is an imprint of the Taylor & Francis Group, an informa business

© 2019 Clare E. Milner

First edition published by Routledge 2008

Library of Congress Cataloging-in-Publication Data
A catalog record has been requested for this book

ISBN: 978-1-138-54123-8 (hbk)
ISBN: 978-0-367-15056-3 (pbk)
ISBN: 978-0-429-20106-6 (ebk)

Typeset in Sabon and Humanist 521
by Servis Filmsetting Ltd, Stockport, Cheshire

To KVJ, for everything

Contents

Figures

Tables

Fundamentals

A to Z Entries

Hot Topics

In Sports

Acknowledgements

Many thanks to the staff at Routledge for inviting me to develop a second edition of this text. I appreciate the efforts of the reviewers who suggested updates to the first edition, particularly the inclusion of the new 'In sports' entries, which use current sports biomechanics research to demonstrate the importance of functional anatomy within kinesiology.

Introduction

This A to Z guide is intended to provide a quick and easily accessible reference for students of musculoskeletal anatomy. It is an appropriate supplement to the traditional anatomy textbook in undergraduate courses, such as applied anatomy, functional anatomy, and kinesiology. Given the applied focus of the subject matter, details of common sports injuries and current hot topics in sports are included alongside the purely anatomical descriptions of each region. The book makes comprehensive reference information available in a concise and easily accessible format. Relevant information about musculoskeletal anatomy can be located quickly and easily without searching through a traditional anatomy textbook that includes details of all of the systems of the body. The compact format of the textbook and the A to Z arrangement of entries enable topics of interest to be located quickly and easily.

Entries are grouped by major joint and include a general introduction to the region, plus detailed descriptions of the bones, joints, ligaments, and muscles. The bones of each joint are illustrated in a detailed figure, including several views to ensure all of the key bony landmarks are shown. These landmarks tie in with the descriptions of ligaments and muscles and their attachments to the bone. New in this edition are figures which illustrate the ligaments at the major joints. The figure labels are lined up on the left and right sides of the diagram. This arrangement is a study tool which enables the labels to be easily covered and then revealed one by one. In this way the figures can be used to test your knowledge of the bones and their landmarks. New tables list the major muscle groups and their action at each joint. The focus of the book is on joints that are involved in movement, including joints of the extremities, vertebral column, and thoracic cage.

Key terminology and essential background information, such as the anatomical planes and axes, are also described in the Fundamentals section located before the A to Z entries.

The A to Z entries are cross-referenced extensively throughout the text to guide the reader to related information about the region of interest. Further reading suggestions are also provided, where appropriate. These direct the reader to both textbooks and selected research articles. In addition, there are Hot Topics boxes which provide further information about contemporary items of interest related to musculoskeletal anatomy and function, such as wearable activity trackers. New in this edition are In Sports entries which provide a more in-depth look at common athletic injuries from a musculoskeletal anatomy perspective.

Fundamentals

Readers who will benefit from a review of the basic terminology and concepts of musculoskeletal anatomy will find this section a good place to start. Familiarity with these fundamentals will facilitate the reader's understanding of the entries describing the different regions of the body.

Anatomical Position

The anatomical position is the reference position of the body that is used when describing movements of the parts of the body (Figure 1). This ensures that movement terminology is consistent, since all axes of rotation (see **planes and axes of movement**) are aligned consistently throughout the upper and lower body. The position is standing upright with the head and feet pointing directly forwards, eyes looking straight ahead. The lower limbs are close together with the feet parallel. The upper limbs are down at the sides of the body with the palms of the hands facing forwards. This position of the upper limbs is different to their natural position during relaxed standing, in which the palms face the body. However, with the upper limbs in the palms-forward position, the flexion-extension axes of the elbow, wrist and joints of the hand are aligned mediolaterally. This puts them in the same orientation as the flexion-extension axes of the other joints of the body. Similarly, the abduction-adduction and internal-external rotation axes are also aligned with the rest of the body. Even though the upper limb may move to a position very different to the anatomical position, the naming of the joint rotations remains the same as in the anatomical position. When interpreting the component parts of a complex upper body movement, it can be helpful to imagine moving the limb back to the anatomical position. It will then be easier to isolate the individual joint movements and identify the axis of rotation and direction of movement.

See also: **anatomical terminology; planes and axes of movement.**

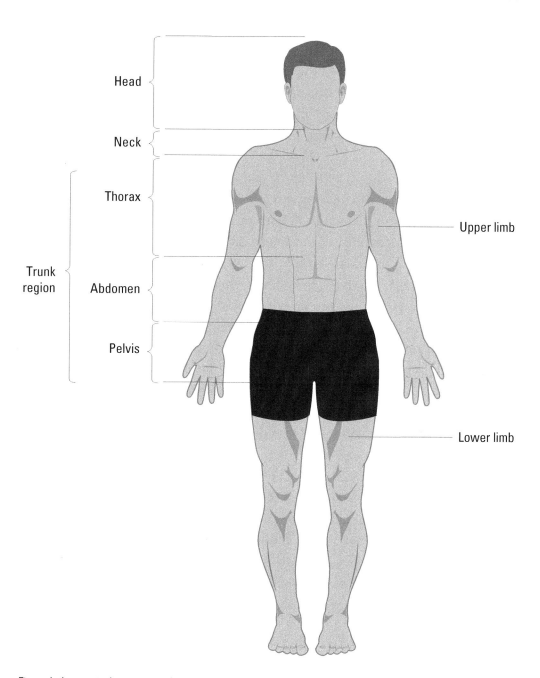

Figure 1 Anatomical position and regions of the body

Anatomical Terminology

When referring to movements of the body or locations of anatomical structures in the body, specific terminology is used. The **planes and axes of movement** are used to describe movements meaningfully and unambiguously. However, the relative locations of parts of the body with respect to the whole also need to be described unambiguously.

The relative location of a point on the **axial skeleton** or **appendicular skeleton** is indicated by the use of either proximal or distal. A point in the appendicular skeleton that is more proximal lies closer to the axial skeleton than one that is more distal on the extremity. For example, the elbow lies proximal to the wrist. Similarly, a point in the axial skeleton that is more cranial is closer to the head than one that is caudal to it. So, the sternum (breastbone) is cranial to the pelvis. Superior and inferior are used to describe points that are above and below each other, respectively. For example, the head is superior to the neck. Whether a point is on the front or the back of the body or a segment is indicated by the use of anterior and posterior respectively, for example, the anterior and posterior heads of the deltoid muscle (see **shoulder complex – muscles**). Ventral and dorsal are alternative anatomical terms for the front and the back of the body, such that the pectoral (chest) muscles lie ventrally on the thorax, and the trapezius muscle lies dorsally on the upper thorax.

To determine on which side of a segment a point lays, medial is used to indicate a point that is closer to the midline of the body, and lateral indicates that a point is further away from the midline. For example, the medial malleolus is the bone on the inside of the ankle, closer to the midline, and the lateral malleolus is the bone on the outside of the ankle, further away from the midline (see **ankle and foot – bones**). Finally, to indicate how close to the centre of a segment a point lies, the terms superficial and deep are used, such that skin is superficial to muscle.

See also: **anatomical position; planes and axes of movement.**

Appendicular Skeleton

The appendicular skeleton consists of the bones of the upper and lower limbs and the shoulder and pelvic girdles, through which the limbs attach to the axial skeleton (Figure 2). The upper limb can be divided into the arm, forearm and hand. Similarly, the lower limb can be divided into the thigh, leg, and foot.

The upper limb bones are the humerus in the arm, the ulna and radius in the forearm, and the carpals, metacarpals, and phalanges of the hand. The shoulder girdle consists of the clavicles (collarbones), which attach to the sternum (breastbone) medially, and the scapulae (shoulder blades). The scapulae are connected to the trunk by muscular attachments only. The major joints of the upper limb are the shoulder, elbow, wrist, and the articulations of the individual digits.

The shoulder is a ball and socket joint. The ball is the proximal end of the humerus, which sits in the shallow socket of the scapula known as the glenoid fossa (see **shoulder complex – joints**). This enables the shoulder to be extremely versatile in its movements and it is capable of multiaxial rotation (see **planes and axes of movement**). The humerus is held in place by strong ligaments and tendinous attachments. The elbow is a hinge joint formed by the articulation of the humerus and ulna and, therefore, has one main axis of rotation for flexion-extension (see **elbow – joints**). The articulation between the radius and the ulna is responsible for pronation and supination of the hand. With the elbow flexed to 90° from the anatomical position, the hand is in a supinated position when it is palm up and pronated when palm down. This movement is achieved by the radius crossing over the ulna in the forearm. The wrist lies between the ulna and radius and the metacarpal bones of the hand. The wrist joint is biaxial, permitting flexion-extension and abduction-adduction (see **wrist and hand – joints**).

The lower limb bones are the femur in the thigh, the patella (kneecap), the tibia (shin bone) and fibula in the calf, and the tarsals, metatarsals, and phalanges in the foot. The pelvic girdle is made up of the hip bones, the os coxae, each of which comprises the ilium, ischium, and pubis. The pelvis is a much more rigid structure than the light and mobile shoulder girdle. The major joints of the lower limb are the hip, knee, ankle, subtalar joint, and the joints of the foot.

There are some similarities between the upper and lower limbs. The hip joint is a ball and socket joint, like the shoulder, but the femur is set more deeply into the hip bone. Comparable to the shoulder, the hip is capable of multiaxial rotation and is the most mobile joint of the lower extremity. When bearing weight, the knee is primarily a hinge joint like the elbow; its major movement is flexion-extension. Only the larger bone of the leg, the tibia, contributes to the knee joint. Both the tibia and fibula contribute to the ankle, along with the talus. The ankle is also a hinge joint: rotation of the foot about the other two axes of rotation is achieved through the oblique subtalar joint of the rear foot.

See also: ankle and foot – bones; axial skeleton; elbow and forearm – bones; hip – bones; knee – bones; shoulder complex – bones; wrist and hand – bones.

AXIAL

APPENDICULAR

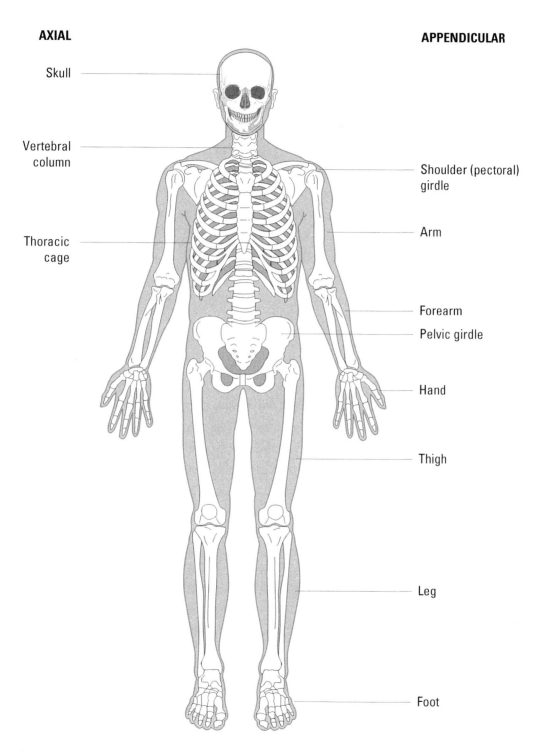

Skull

Vertebral
column

Thoracic
cage

Shoulder (pectoral)
girdle

Arm

Forearm

Pelvic girdle

Hand

Thigh

Leg

Foot

Figure 2 Axial and appendicular skeleton

Articulating Surfaces

Articulating surfaces are the cartilage-covered ends of bone which touch adjacent bones at joints. In synovial joints, these surfaces are covered with articular hyaline cartilage. Hyaline cartilage is flexible and resilient, providing a cushion between the ends of the bones where they come into contact with each other. The cartilage is able to absorb some of the compressive forces at the joint, and so help to protect the bone from damage. Cartilage itself does not contain any blood vessels or nerves. This means that it relies on the fluid which surrounds it (synovial fluid) for nutrients. The compressive forces that occur at the joint as it is loaded help to move these fluids into and out of the cartilage. This happens in a similar way to squeezing a sponge which is submerged in a bowl of water: as the sponge is squeezed, water is forced out, then when the pressure is released, water rushes back into the sponge. This is why it is important to load the joints regularly to keep them healthy.

The primary function of cartilage is to protect the bone from damage by distributing the load over a large surface area, which decreases the stress at any one part of the bone's surface. Articular cartilage also helps to minimize friction between adjacent bones during movement by providing a smooth surface. These two functions of cartilage help to minimize wear and damage to the articular surfaces of the joint. This is an important role because wear and damage to the articulating surfaces are a precursor to the development of osteoarthritis at the joint. This is a painful condition in which the protective cartilage is damaged and wears away, leaving the bones directly in contact with one another. Osteoarthritis is a major cause of reduced mobility in older adults, primarily affecting the knees and hips, which are the major weight-bearing joints in the lower extremities.

See also: ankle and foot – joints; elbow and forearm – joints; head and neck – joints; hip – joint; joint classification; joints; knee – joints; lumbar spine and pelvis – joints; shoulder complex – joints; thoracic region – joints; wrist and hand – joints.

Axial Skeleton

The axial skeleton consists of the vertebral column and skull plus the ribs and associated bones of the thorax. It is the central part of the skeleton and the **appendicular skeleton** attaches to it through the shoulder and pelvic girdles. The vertebral column contains 33 vertebrae in four regions; moving distally from the head, these are the 7 cervical, 12 thoracic, 5 lumbar, 5 sacral, and 4 coccygeal vertebrae. Vertebrae within a region are numbered in ascending order in a proximal to distal direction. The sacrum and coccyx are made up of fused vertebrae, whereas the vertebrae in the other regions are movable. The vertebral column is not simply a stack of vertebrae, but has four curved regions. The cervical curve is convex anteriorly, followed by the thoracic curve, which is concave anteriorly, the anteriorly convex lumbar curve, and the anteriorly concave pelvic curve. Since the vertebrae protect the spinal cord, injuries to this region are potentially very severe. Depending on the vertebral level at which the spinal cord is damaged, more or less of the body may be paralyzed. As a result, most sports have rules that are designed to minimize the risk of spinal cord damage. For example, American football bans tackles made with the head of the tackler as the first point of contact with the opponent. This rule was introduced after changes to protective headgear led to a large increase in cervical spine injuries because of an increase in the use of this tackling technique.

The bones of the thorax (chest) form a protective cage around the major organs of the chest cavity, principally the lungs and heart. Each vertebra of the thoracic region has a pair of ribs associated with it. Of the 12 pairs of ribs, ten are attached to the sternum (breast bone) anteriorly by costal cartilage. The first seven pairs are true ribs attaching directly to the sternum via their own costal cartilage. The next three pairs are the false ribs: they attach to the sternum indirectly via the costal cartilage of the ribs above. The most distal two pairs of ribs are not secured anteriorly and are, therefore, known as floating or free ribs. As the link between the upper and lower body, the bones of the thorax can be subjected to large forces in those sports that call for power to be transferred from one part of the body to another. For example, rib stress fractures are relatively common in rowers. During the rowing stroke, a rower must drive his or her legs against the foot plate of the boat and subsequently transfer the power generated at the feet to the oar handle and propel the boat through the water. For the force developed at the foot plate to be transferred effectively to the oar blade, the trunk must provide a rigid link between the lower and upper body. The muscular tension necessary to achieve this force places great strain on the ribs and may result in a stress fracture. This injury tends to occur during winter training when the rower is training at a lower stroke rate, but generating more force with each stroke.

The skull consists of the cranium, the large dome that houses and protects the brain, and the bones of the face. It is made up of eight cranial and 14 facial bones. All of these, except the mandible or jawbone, are attached rigidly to each other in adults by interlaced articulations called sutures (see **joint classification**). Injuries to the skull in sports tend to be acute trauma from contact with another athlete, equipment, or the ground.

Further Reading

Evans, G., & Redgrave, A. (2016). Great Britain rowing team guideline for diagnosis and management of rib stress injury: Part 1. *British Journal of Sports Medicine, 50,* 266–269.

See also: **appendicular skeleton; head and neck – bones; lumbar spine and pelvis – bones; thoracic region – bones; vertebral structure.**

Bone

Bone is hard, strong and stiff and its function is to support the soft tissues of the body and protect vital organs. It also serves as a storage site for minerals, especially calcium, and is the source of new blood cells. Bone contains calcium carbonate, calcium phosphate, collagen (a flexible fibrous protein), and water. Bone is a living tissue with living cells and it is constantly being remodelled in response to the current stresses and strains that are being applied to it.

There are two types of bone, which are classified by their porosity. The greater the volume of mineralized (calcified) tissue in the bone, the less porous it is. Cortical or compact bone has more than 70 per cent mineralized tissue by volume. This type of bone is the outside layer of bone. The bone type on the inside of a bone is more porous and is called trabecular or cancellous or spongy bone. Spongy is also a good way to describe its structure. The mineralized bone tissue forms a honeycomb structure with lots of pockets or spaces in it. The structure of trabecular bone makes bones more lightweight. The pattern of the mineralized part of the trabecular bone develops in response to the stress patterns that the bone is subjected to, with more tissue laid down in areas of high stress. This allows bone to be both light and strong. Although cortical bone looks solid, it has bone cells within it, plus channels for blood and lymph vessels and nerves throughout its structure. It should be noted that the whole of the inside of long bones is not filled with trabecular bone. The central medullary cavity down the shaft, or diaphysis, of a long bone is filled with bone marrow. This is the site of new blood cell production. Trabecular bone is only laid down at the expanded ends of long bones (the epiphyses), where it adds strength to the bone's structure in areas of high stress.

See also: ankle and foot – bones; appendicular skeleton; articulating surfaces; axial skeleton; bone classification; bony landmarks; elbow and forearm – bones; head and neck – bones; hip – bones; knee – bones; lumbar spine and pelvis – bones; shoulder complex – bones; thoracic region – bones.

Bone Classification

Bones can be classified according to their structure and shape. There are five categories of bone when classified by structure: long bones, short bones, flat bones, sesamoid bones and irregular bones. Long bones are those which are basically tubular and have a long shaft. A good example is the femur in the thigh. However, the classification does not refer to the actual length of the bones; a long bone is simply longer than it is wide, like a narrow tube. The phalanges, metacarpals and metatarsals in the hands (see **wrist and hand – bones**) and feet (see **ankle and foot – bones**) are also long bones, even though they are quite small.

Short bones are those with a cuboidal shape, with width about equal to length. The tarsal and carpal bones in the feet and wrists are short bones.

Flat bones are thin and flattened and typically play a protective role. They are usually curved surfaces, not flat as the name suggests. The bones of the skull (see **head and neck – bones**) and the pelvis (see **lumbar spine and pelvis**) are flat bones, as well as the ribs, scapula and sternum (see **thoracic region – bones**).

Sesamoid bones are a special category of bones that are embedded within a tendon. They are sometimes considered to be a sub-category of short bones. The best example of a sesamoid bone is the patella (kneecap), which lies within the tendon of the quadriceps muscle at the knee (see **knee – bones**). The patella keeps the tendon further away from the joint, which changes the angle of the tendon and enables the quadriceps muscle to produce more torque to move the joint. The pisiform in the wrist is also a sesamoid bone. There are also two small sesamoid bones under the first metatarsal head in the foot, which help to protect the tendons from damage when the foot is on the ground. Sesamoid bones vary in size and shape between people and an individual may have other sesamoid bones in addition to those described.

The final category is irregular bones. Irregular bones are those which do not fit into any of the other categories! The vertebrae of the spine are irregular bones (see **vertebral structure**).

See also: ankle and foot – bones; appendicular skeleton; articulating surfaces; axial skeleton; bone; bony landmarks; elbow and forearm – bones; head and neck – bones; hip – bones; knee – bones; lumbar spine and pelvis – bones; shoulder complex – bones; thoracic region – bones.

Bony Landmarks

Bones have many different landmarks or features at and around the joints. Bony landmarks can be divided into articulating and non-articulating surfaces. **Articulating surfaces** are smooth cartilage-covered parts of bone that are part of the joints. Non-articulating surfaces are located at various sites on the bone where muscles, tendons, and ligaments attach. A head is an articulating surface that is rounded like a ball. The head of the humerus and the head of the femur are part of ball and socket joints at the shoulder (see **shoulder complex – bones**) and hip (see **hip – bones**) respectively. A condyle is a large articulating knob that is part of a compound joint. Examples are the femoral condyles at the knee (see **knee – bones**). A facet is a flat or shallow articular surface found at a gliding or sliding joint (see **joint classification**). The facets of the superior and inferior articular processes of the vertebrae are good examples (see **vertebral structure**).

Non-articulating surfaces for the attachment of ligaments and tendons include large rough processes called tuberosities, such as the tibial tuberosity for the attachment of the tendon of quadriceps (see **knee – bones**). A small rounded process is known as a tubercle, such as the greater and lesser tubercles of the proximal humerus (see **shoulder complex – bones**). A process is a bony prominence, like the xiphoid process on the distal end of the sternum (see **thoracic region – bones**). A spine is a sharp process, such as the anterior superior iliac spine of the pelvis (see **lumbar spine and pelvis – bones**). An epicondyle is a projection above a condyle, such as the lateral and medial epicondyles of the femur (see **knee – bones**). There are two kinds of depression found on the bones: a shallow depression called a fossa and a small pit called a fovea. Examples are the iliac fossa of the pelvis (see **lumbar spine and pelvis – bones**) and the fovea capitis of the head of the femur (see **hip – bones**). There are various holes through the bones, known as foramina. For example, every vertebra has a vertebral foramen for the spinal cord to pass through (see **vertebral structure**).

See also: **anatomical terminology; appendicular skeleton; axial skeleton; bone.**

Joint Classification

Joints can be classified according to their structure or function. Classifying joints by structure, there are three major categories: fibrous, cartilaginous and synovial. There are three subtypes of fibrous joint: sutures, syndesmoses and gomphoses, and two subtypes of cartilaginous joint: synchondroses and symphyses. Fibrous joints are those in which the articulating bones are connected by fibrous connective tissue. There is no joint space or cavity and the joint is either immovable or only slightly movable. The three subtypes of fibrous joints differ in the types of articulation that they make. Sutures are found where the bones of the skull come together. They are the wavy interlocking edges of the skull bones (see **head and neck – bones**). The skull is made up of several interlocking bones, which allows for skull growth during childhood when the bones are still separate. The bones are tightly bound together by fibrous connective tissue and minimal movement occurs between them. The primary role of the bones of the skull is to protect the brain. The individual bones eventually fuse together during middle age. A gomphosis is another specialized type of fibrous joint. It is a peg-in-socket type of articulation, with the roots of the teeth being the pegs and the jaw bones containing the sockets. The periodontal ligament holds the tooth in the jaw bone and movement is minimal. The third type of fibrous joint is a syndesmosis, and is simply two bones connected by ligaments. The amount of movement possible at this type of joint depends on the length of the ligament. For example, the inferior anterior tibiofibular ligament, between the two leg bones just above the ankle, is short and only a small amount of 'give' is possible between the bones (see **ankle and foot – ligaments**). In contrast, the interosseous membrane in the forearm has longer fibres which allow free movement between the radius and ulna as the forearm pronates and supinates (see **elbow and forearm – joints**).

Cartilaginous joints are those in which the articulating bones are connected by cartilage. They do not have a joint cavity. The amount of movement possible at cartilaginous joints varies from immovable to highly movable, with synchondroses being immovable and symphyses being slightly or highly movable. A synchondrosis is a joint where the bones are firmly connected by hyaline cartilage (see **articulating surfaces**). Examples include the epiphyseal (growth) plates in the long bones of the extremities and sternocostal synchondroses between the sternum (breastbone) and the anterior end of the ribs in the thoracic cage (see thoracic region – joints). The second type of cartilaginous joint is a symphysis, in which the bones are connected by fibrocartilage. In these joints, hyaline cartilage is present on the articulating parts of the bone. These joints are somewhat movable and include the intervertebral joints. The fibrocartilaginous intervertebral disc connects the vertebral bodies and acts as a shock absorber within the vertebral column (see **thoracic region – joints**). Another example is the pubic symphysis on the anterior aspect of the pelvis (see **lumbar spine and pelvis – bones**). This joint becomes quite flexible prior to childbirth to enable the infant to pass more easily through the birth canal.

The third type of joint is a synovial joint. In this joint, articular cartilage is present on the bony surfaces, the bones are connected by ligaments and the joint is surrounded by a joint capsule. This type of joint is the most movable and is the most common type of joint, especially in the limbs. Examples of synovial joints include the knee, hip and elbow joints.

Joints can also be categorized according to their function. There is some overlap here with the divisions according to structure. Synarthrodial joints are immovable and include sutures and gomphoses. Amphiarthrodial joints are slightly movable and include syndesmoses and synchondroses. Diarthrodial joints are freely movable and equate to synovial joints.

See also: **ankle and foot – joints; articulating surfaces; elbow and forearm – joints; head and neck – joints; hip – joint; joints; knee – joints; lumbar spine and pelvis – joints; shoulder complex – joints; thoracic region – joints; wrist and hand – joints.**

Joints

Joints are also known as articulations. A joint is the junction between two or more bones. Typically, joints are found at the ends of long bones. In short and irregular bones, joints are found wherever a bone touches another bone. The primary function of joints is to permit movement between the adjacent bones. However, not all joints are movable. The amount of movement possible at a joint varies from it being freely movable, to only a small amount of movement, to no movement whatsoever between adjacent bones (see **joint classification**).

The freely movable synovial (diarthrodial) joints can be classified according to their structure. At the simplest level, synovial joints fit into one of two groups: simple or compound. A simple joint has only two **articulating surfaces**, one on each of the two bones that are touching. Compound joints have more than two articulating surfaces. For example, at the knee (tibiofemoral joint) there are four articulating surfaces on two bones. At the elbow, three bones articulate with each other. Synovial joints can also be classified according to the shapes of the articulating surfaces. There are six different types of synovial joint according to their shape: ball and socket, gliding, ellipsoidal, hinge, saddle and pivot joints.

A ball and socket (enarthrodial) joint consists of a bone with a ball-shaped head that sits in a cup-shaped cavity. This type of joint is highly mobile and allows movement about all three axes (see **planes and axes of movement**). Examples are the hip and shoulder joints. The hip has a deep socket and good bony stability, whereas the shoulder (glenohumeral) joint has a large ball and shallow socket. This gives it less bony stability, but allows a greater range of motion.

Ellipsoidal (condyloidal) joints consist of a bone with an oval articular surface and a bone with an oval cavity. This type of joint is biaxial, allowing movement about two of the three axes. No rotation is possible about the long axis of the bone in this case. Examples include the wrist complex and the metacarpophalangeal joints (knuckles).

Another type of biaxial joint is a saddle (sellar) joint. In this case, each joint has perpendicular concave and convex areas, like a horse saddle. Again, there is no rotation about the long axis in this joint. This type of joint is less common than the ellipsoidal joint; the first carpometacarpal joint is an example.

A hinge joint is found between a bone with a cylindrical articular surface and a bone with a trough-shaped cavity. This joint is uniaxial, allowing movement about only one axis. Movement at this joint is planar (i.e. occurs in only one plane – that perpendicular to the axis of rotation). Examples include the ankle (talocrural), elbow (ulnohumeral) and finger (interphalangeal) joints.

A pivot (trochoidal) joint is a special type of uniaxial joint. In this case, a bone with a rounded end is encircled by a ring formed from the second bone and its ligament: rotation is possible about the long axis of the encircled bone only. Pivot joints in the body are the proximal radioulnar and atlantoaxial joints.

The least mobile type of synovial joint is a gliding (arthrodial) joint. This joint has flat articular surfaces and only allows short gliding or sliding movements between them. Examples include intervertebral, intertarsal and intercarpal joints.

See also: **ankle and foot – joints; articulating surfaces; elbow and forearm – joints; head and neck – joints; hip – joint; joint classification; knee – joints; lumbar spine and pelvis – joints; thoracic region – joints; wrist and hand – joints.**

Ligaments

Ligaments are soft tissue structures which connect bone to bone at a joint. They are generally inelastic, and their major role is to prevent excessive joint motion. When the ligament is pulled tight by movement of the bones, it prevents further movement. In this way ligaments contribute to joint stability. Although they cannot be stretched much, ligaments are flexible. They can be thought of as a short piece of string connecting two bones, which can move with the bones until it is pulled tight, when it resists further movement in that direction. Ligaments are composed mainly of collagen fibres, which are inelastic. Other components include water, fibroblast cells, ground substance and elastin. Most ligaments contain only a very small amount of elastin, which is an elastic fibre. However, there is a spinal ligament with special elastic properties which contains twice as much elastin as collagen. This yellow-coloured ligament is called the ligamentum flavum and it runs the length of the vertebral column. It plays an important role in spinal stability. This ligament is stretched when the trunk is flexed and recoils when the trunk extends from the flexed position. This elastic recoil assists with the extension movement of the trunk (see **thoracic region – ligaments**).

Excessive torque at a joint can rupture a ligament. Common examples of ligament rupture include rolling or spraining an ankle, when the foot inverts excessively and ligaments on the lateral side of the ankle are torn (see **In Sports 1**), and anterior cruciate ligament rupture (see **In Sports 2**). Since ligaments do not have a very good blood supply, healing can be slow and the ligament may take a long time to return to its original strength. Once a ligament injury has occurred, it is common to injure the same tissue again in the future.

See also: **ankle and foot – ligaments; elbow and forearm – ligaments; head and neck – ligaments; hip – ligaments; knee – ligaments; lumbar spine and pelvis – ligaments; shoulder complex – ligaments; thoracic region – ligaments; wrist and hand – ligaments.**

Muscle

Muscles are the contractile tissues of the body. They can move body parts or alter the shape of the internal organs. Muscle cells are specialized to enable them to contract and generate force (see **skeletal muscle – structure**). The individual cells are long and narrow and are referred to as muscle fibres. There are three types of muscle in the body, each with its own specialized activity. Skeletal muscle moves the bones at the joints and is under voluntary control via the somatic nervous system and can be activated at will. This type of muscle is most important in functional anatomy and is covered in detail in its own section.

The other two types of muscles are involuntary, meaning that they are controlled by the autonomic nervous system and cannot be activated at will. Cardiac muscle is found in the walls of the heart and the great vessels. Smooth muscle is found in the walls of most blood vessels and hollow organs such as the intestine. Cardiac muscle forms the myocardium, the muscular wall of the heart. It is also found in the walls of the aorta, pulmonary vein and superior vena cava. Contractions of the cardiac muscle make the heart beat. Heart rate is controlled by the autonomic nervous system via specialized pacemaker cells. Cardiac muscle does not fatigue and contracts and relaxes continuously day and night for many years. Smooth muscle is found in the walls of most blood vessels, parts of the digestive tract, hair follicles and in the eye. This type of involuntary muscle can remain partially contracted for long periods of time. For example, smooth muscle controls the thickness of the lens of the eye by squeezing it, enabling the eye to focus at different distances.

See also: ankle and foot – muscles; elbow and forearm – muscles; head and neck – muscles; hip – muscles; knee – muscles; lumbar spine and pelvis – muscles; muscle contraction – types; shoulder complex – muscles; skeletal muscle classification; skeletal muscle function; skeletal muscle structure; thoracic region – muscles; wrist and hand – muscles.

Planes and Axes of Movement

There are three cardinal planes and three axes about which joint movement can occur. A plane is two-dimensional, like a page in a book or an image on a television screen. The only movement that can be clearly seen in a plane is one in which the body segments move within that plane. That is, they do not move towards or away from the plane, but within its two-dimensional space. In the following examples, assume that the person is standing in the **anatomical position**. The sagittal plane is the one seen when looking from the side (Figure 3). If you look at a person from the side, you can clearly see the movement of flexing and extending the knee. Knee flexion and extension occur in the sagittal plane. The angle between the leg and thigh can be seen increasing and decreasing as the knee extends and flexes. However, abduction and adduction of the hip cannot be clearly seen in the sagittal plane. The changing angle between the thigh and pelvis cannot be seen from the sagittal, or side, view. Hip abduction and adduction can be clearly seen if you look at the person from the front; this is the frontal, or coronal, plane. In addition to the sagittal and frontal planes, there is a horizontal plane, the transverse plane, which is seen when looking down on a person from above. Internal and external rotation movements of the body segments can be seen in this plane, such as internal and external rotation of the hip.

All joint movements can be considered to be rotations about an axis, like a door moving around the pins of its hinges, as one segment rotates about the other. There are three anatomical axes which are associated with the three cardinal planes. The flexion-extension movement that can be seen in the sagittal plane is rotation about a mediolateral axis. This axis lies parallel to the frontal plane and perpendicular to the sagittal plane. It runs from side-to-side across the joint and is occasionally referred to as the frontal axis. The abduction-adduction movement in the frontal plane is rotation about an anteroposterior axis. This axis lies parallel to the sagittal plane and perpendicular to the frontal plane and is occasionally called the sagittal axis. Third, internal and external rotations are about a vertical axis. This axis is parallel to both the frontal and sagittal planes and perpendicular to the transverse plane. It is also referred to as the longitudinal, or long, axis.

See also: **anatomical position, anatomical terminology.**

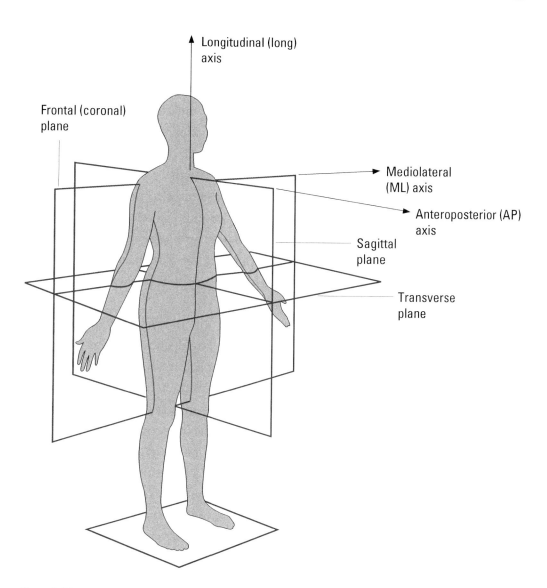

Longitudinal (long)
axis

Frontal (coronal)
plane

Mediolateral
(ML) axis

Anteroposterior (AP)
axis

Sagittal
plane

Transverse
plane

Figure 3 Planes and axes of movement

Skeletal Muscle – Classification

Muscles are organized into groups within body segments. These groups are separated by fascia (fibrous connective tissue) into individual compartments. For example, in the upper extremity, there are three arm muscle groups: the shoulder girdle, the posterior arm and the anterior arm muscles. Similarly, in the lower extremity, there are anterior, medial and posterior thigh compartments.

Muscle names are derived from characteristics of where the muscle is found and what it does. Naming conventions include references to the location, shape, relative size and direction of fibres, number of origins, location of attachments and the action of the muscle. They are often relative terms, comparing one muscle to another within the same segment. Understanding the classification of a muscle described by its name reveals important information about its location, structure and function.

Muscles may be named according to their location and the body part they are associated with. Internal and external refers to being deeper or more superficial respectively, for example, internal and external obliques on the trunk. Anterior and posterior describe the muscle's position relative to a bone, such as tibialis anterior and posterior in the leg (see **ankle and foot – muscles**). Muscle names may explicitly include the names of body parts, such as the intercostal muscles between the ribs (costa = rib: see **thoracic region – muscles**) or the arm muscle brachialis (brachium = arm: see **elbow and forearm – muscles**). The overall shape of the muscle may be incorporated into the name: deltoid is triangular in shape (the symbol for the Greek letter delta is a triangle: see **shoulder complex – muscles**). Relative size is often used in naming muscles within a group. The gluteals are a good example, named from largest to smallest as gluteus maximus, medius and minimus (see **lumbar spine and pelvis – muscles**). Pairs of muscles which are similar, with one being longer than the other (including the length of its tendon) are named as longus and brevis (long and short): for example, peroneus longus and brevis in the lower extremity (see **ankle and foot – muscles**). The direction in which the fibres of the muscle run can also be incorporated into the name. There are several good examples in the abdomen (see **lumbar spine and pelvis – muscles**). Transversus abdominis has fibres running perpendicular to the midline, horizontally (in the transverse plane) around the abdomen. The fibres of the oblique muscles are at an oblique angle to the midline, running diagonally across the abdomen.

The number of origins, or heads, may be incorporated into the name as 'ceps'. Biceps brachii, triceps brachii and quadriceps femoris have two, three and four heads respectively. Muscles may be named by the location of their origin and insertion attachments, with the origin being named first, for example, brachioradialis originates on the arm (brachium) and inserts onto the radius. The action of the muscle may be incorporated into its name as flexor, extensor, adductor or abductor. Adductor longus adducts the thigh at the hip (see **hip – muscles**). Muscle names may become quite long if they include a combination of these different classifications: extensor carpi radialis longus is a long wrist (carpi) extensor on the radial side of the forearm (see **wrist and hand – muscles**). This name incorporates the action, joint, location and relative size of the muscle.

See also: **head and neck – muscles; hip – muscles; knee – muscles; muscle; muscle contraction – types; skeletal muscle – function; skeletal muscle – structure.**

Skeletal Muscle Contraction – Types

There are several different types of skeletal muscle contraction, which result in different movement patterns at the joint that the muscle crosses. In a concentric contraction, the muscle shortens under tension. The direction of movement at the joint is in the same direction as the muscle torque being generated. A concentric contraction is what is typically thought of when one refers to 'flexing' a muscle; for example, concentric contraction of the biceps brachii (located anteriorly on the arm) results in elbow flexion, such as during a curl exercise holding a weight in the hand. Eccentric contraction is the opposite of concentric contraction. In this case, the muscle lengthens under tension and the joint movement is in the opposite direction to the torque generated. Typically, eccentric contraction counteracts the action of gravity on the joint and slows down joint movement. Using the example of the biceps curl exercise at the elbow again, the elbow joint will move from flexion into extension with eccentric contraction of the biceps. The action of gravity would naturally pull the weight downwards, moving the elbow into extension from the flexed position without any muscle action needed. The eccentric contraction of biceps counteracts gravity and allows the weight to be lowered slowly and under control to the extended position of the elbow.

A third type of contraction is isometric, in which the muscle is under tension, but the joint does not move. In this case, there are two opposing torques which cancel each other out. The 'iso' part of the name means 'the same' and the 'metric' part refers to length. That is, the muscle stays the same length (compared to shortening in concentric and lengthening in eccentric contraction). In this case, there is typically a pair of muscles working against each other to keep the joint fixed in position. This pair of muscles is referred to as an agonist-antagonist pair. For example, to keep the elbow joint in a fixed position, the biceps and triceps would form an agonist-antagonist pair, since one is an elbow flexor and the other an elbow extensor. Isometric contraction is found in strength training and other activities when a joint needs to be fixed in position to provide stability while movement occurs at another joint. For example, the fixed position of the elbow while the shoulder abducts during a lateral dumbbell raise.

There are two more types of muscle contraction which are special cases of concentric and eccentric contractions: isokinetic and isotonic. In an isokinetic muscle contraction, there is a constant speed of rotation of the joint. This type of movement is utilized in a rehabilitation setting, where an isokinetic dynamometer machine is used to restrict the joint motion to a fixed speed. An isotonic muscle contraction is one in which the amount of muscle tension or tone is kept constant. Since the effectiveness of a muscle in moving a joint may change depending on the angular position of the joint, the amount of muscle tension required to lift a weight may change at different stages of the movement. This is related to the line of action of the muscle across the joint and how close to the joint centre it passes. Strength training machines are often designed to create isotonic contractions during weight-lifting exercises. For example, an arm curl machine is typically designed with a cam-shaped pulley for the cable to pass over between the joint and the weight stack, rather than a round pulley. The changing curvature of the cam pulley is designed to alter the resistance of the machine at different stages of the arm curl to keep the muscle tension constant, and the contraction isotonic. The rationale for this is that muscle strength will be evenly developed throughout the range of motion of the exercise. With traditional free weights, more muscle force is required at some stages of the movement than others, and the body develops in response to this.

See also: **muscle; skeletal muscle – classification; skeletal muscle – function; skeletal muscle – structure.**

Skeletal Muscle – Function

Skeletal muscle is voluntary muscle. Its primary function is to move the body at the joints. Skeletal muscle typically makes up about 40 per cent of body weight and there are more than 600 skeletal muscles in the body. Skeletal muscle has four major functions: movement, posture, joint stabilization and heat generation. Skeletal muscle is attached to the bones of the skeleton via connective tissue (see **skeletal muscle – structure**). The origin and insertion of a muscle are on different bones, with the muscle (or its tendon) crossing one or more joints. When the muscle contracts and shortens, it moves the bone at the joint the muscle crosses; coordinated movement of bones by muscles moves the whole body. Muscles which cross only one joint are known as 'monoarticular' muscles. For example, the vasti muscles, which are part of the quadriceps femoris, are monoarticular knee extensors. Their origin is on the femur and insertion on the tibia with the muscle tendon crossing the front of the knee. Muscles which cross two joints are 'biarticular' and can move either one or both joints depending on the action of the surrounding muscles. For example, rectus femoris is the fourth of the quadriceps muscles and it crosses the front of both the hip and knee joints. Rectus femoris can both flex the hip and extend the knee. Either of these actions can be held in check by the antagonist muscle group. For example, if hip extensors oppose the hip flexion action of rectus femoris, it will only extend the knee during concentric contraction.

Skeletal muscles also maintain body posture. Periodic contraction of the muscles enables the body to remain in a standing or sitting position. In addition to actively moving the joints, muscles are also involved in joint stabilization. A low level of muscle tone, in which the muscle is kept at a constant low level of contraction keeps tension on the muscle tendon and helps to stabilize the joint. This is especially important at joints like the shoulder and knee which do not get much stability from their bone structure. Finally, muscular contraction generates heat. Heat generation by muscles helps the body to maintain its normal temperature of 98.6°F (37°C).

See also: **muscle; muscle contraction – types; skeletal muscle – classification; skeletal muscle – structure.**

Skeletal Muscle – Structure

Skeletal muscle consists of muscle fibres (cells), connective tissue, blood vessels and nerves; it is surrounded by epimysium (sheath of connective tissue: epi = outside, myo = muscle). Within the muscle, bundles of muscle fibres are surrounded by perimysium (peri = around) and referred to as muscle fascicles. The individual muscle fibre is a single muscle cell and is surrounded by endomysium (endo = within). All of the connective tissue sheaths are continuous with the muscle tendons. Skeletal muscle can have either a direct or indirect attachment to bone. The most common indirect attachment is via a tendon, which is connective tissue that extends beyond the muscle. Tendons are rope-like cords which attach to bones at raised areas such as tubercles, tuberosities, processes and spines (see **bony landmarks**). An aponeurosis is a flat sheet of connective tissue. A good example is the external oblique aponeurosis on the abdomen (see **lumbar spine and pelvis – muscles**). Muscles can also be attached directly to bones via short strands of connective tissue. These are referred to as direct or fleshy attachments.

Muscle fibres are highly specialized cells. They contain multiple cell nuclei because they come from the fusion of many individual cells during embryonic development. The fibres are long cylindrical cells which are up to 100 microns in diameter (about 10 times greater than a typical cell) and tens of centimetres long. The microscopic structure of muscle fibres gives them a striped or striated appearance, hence the alternative name for skeletal muscle: striated muscle. Muscle fibres contain two types of muscle filament which slide over each other in contraction, thus shortening the muscle. The thick filaments consist of actin and ATPase (an enzyme that releases energy for the contraction). The thin filaments are actin. The filaments run in alternating parallel rows of thick and thin filaments along the length of the muscle fibre, with the ends of each row of fibres overlapping the ends of the next row. The pattern of striations on the muscle cell corresponds to the actin (I band) and myosin (A band) filament location, and the overlap between them (Figure 4). The H zone is the central part of the A band which is not overlapped with the actin filaments. The I band consists only of actin filaments. The M line is found in the middle of the H zone and runs perpendicular to the myosin filaments. The Z line is found running perpendicular to the rows of filaments in the middle of the actin filaments. The segment between adjacent Z lines is called a sarcomere; it is the basic unit of contraction. A myofibril is a row of many sarcomeres. The striations in adjacent myofibrils are aligned, thus the banding can be seen in the whole muscle fibre as stripes.

Force is generated by muscle contraction and is explained by the sliding filament theory. At each end of the thick filaments is a cross-bridge (myosin head), which attaches to the adjacent thin filament at each end of the sarcomere. The cross-bridge pulls the thin filament towards the centre of the sarcomere by swivelling inwards. It then releases the thin filament and returns to its original position, where it reattaches to the thin filament further along its length. The process repeats many times over during a contraction and the filaments slide over each other. The action of the cross-bridge can be likened to pulling in a rope hand over hand.

See also: **muscle; muscle contraction – types; skeletal muscle – classification; skeletal muscle – function.**

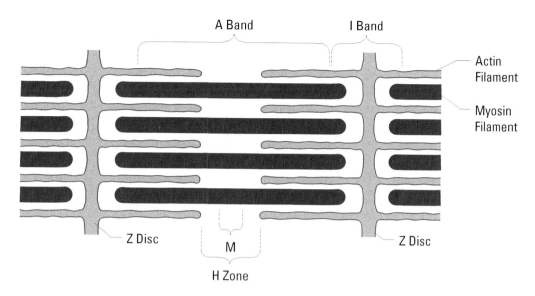

Figure 4 Skeletal muscle structure. Adapted from Watkins (2014).

A to Z Entries

Ankle and Foot

The ankle and foot form a complex region containing many joints, which provide flexibility and enable the foot to adapt to its environment. This flexibility of the foot is essential because it is the point of contact between the ground and the body; it must be able to adapt to changes in terrain with minimum perturbation of the body system as a whole. The many bones and joints in the foot enable it to play multiple roles during activity; it is a flexible shock-attenuating structure during the early part of the stance phase of walking, and then becomes a rigid lever during push-off at the end of the stance phase. This change in dynamic function is achieved by activity of the invertor and evertor muscles of the foot (see **ankle and foot – muscles**). The invertors rotate the foot about its longitudinal axis from a flexible pronated position to a rigid supinated position and the evertors move the foot in the opposite direction (see **ankle and foot – joints**).

Owing to the foot's position as the most distal segment in the body, the ankle and foot region is subjected to high loads, particularly during running and jumping activities. It is also subjected to large shear forces during cutting and other side-step activities that occur in sports. As a result of these high loads and extreme positions, the ankle and foot are at high risk of injury (see **In Sports 1**). Additionally, injuries related to ankle and foot risk factors may manifest themselves higher up the kinetic chain – in the leg, knee, or hip. Overuse injuries related to foot and ankle structure and mechanics include plantar fasciitis, patellofemoral pain, and tibial stress fractures (see **Hot Topic 1**).

See also: ankle and foot – bones; ankle and foot – joints; ankle and foot – ligaments; ankle and foot – muscles; appendicular skeleton; foot arches.

Hot Topic 1 Tibial Stress Fracture in Runners

Stress fractures are a common overuse injury in runners. The most common site of a stress fracture is the tibia, typically in the region about a third of the way up the bone from the ankle. Female runners are at higher risk of tibial stress fracture than male runners, although it is unclear what the root cause of the difference is. A stress fracture develops when microscopic damage that is done to the bone during repeated loading accumulates over time. In runners, the bones are loaded every time the foot hits the ground. Bone constantly repairs itself and, in the healthy runner, the rate of repair or remodelling of the bone keeps pace with the rate of microdamage. This enables the bone to remain healthy and even become stronger over time to better withstand the repeated pavement pounding. However, if the balance is tipped and the rate of damage exceeds the rate of repair, microcracks in the bone eventually join up and a stress fracture occurs. A runner takes about 500 steps on each foot during every mile of running, each step subjects the body to a peak force of about three times the body's weight. It is easy to appreciate the huge cumulative load experienced by the lower limbs over a period of weeks or months of running.

Numerous factors contribute to the development of a stress fracture and can tip the balance between damage and repair. Some of these can be modified to try and reduce the risk of injury. Structural factors such as the shape of the bone may predispose some runners to injury, but these cannot be altered. External factors related to training may also contribute and these can be altered to reduce the risk of injury. For example, the training programme may be a cause of injury if the weekly mileage (the total load on the body) is increased too quickly and tips the balance between damage and repair of the bone. Poor nutrition can also weaken the bone and reduce bone density, lowering the threshold at which loading will lead to stress fracture. This is a special concern among competitive distance runners who diet to reduce their body weight as much as possible and so restrict their intake of essential nutrients. The biomechanics of running (running technique), may also be an important factor. For example, some runners tend to hit the ground harder with every step, even after differences in weight are taken into consideration. These runners will have a higher total load on the body for every mile of running compared to those who are lighter on their feet.

After a tibial stress fracture, a period of rest and rehabilitation of up to 12 weeks is needed to allow the bone to remodel and repair itself. After sustaining a stress fracture once, the runner is quite likely to get another stress fracture in the future if they keep doing the same things they were before the injury. To avoid another stress fracture, special attention should be paid to factors such as the training programme, nutrition, and running biomechanics to correct any deficiencies which may put the athlete at increased risk of injury.

Further Reading

Warden, S. J., Davis, I. S. & Fredericson, M. (2014). Management and prevention of bone stress injuries in long-distance runners. *Journal of Orthopaedic and Sports Physical Therapy, 44*, 749–765.

In Sports I Chronic Ankle Instability

Ankle sprains or 'rolling an ankle' are a common injury in many sports. While either the medial or lateral ankle ligaments may be damaged, depending on the position of the foot and ankle at the time of injury, lateral ankle sprains are by far the most common. The injury occurs when the foot is forcibly supinated. The lateral ankle ligaments become taut in this position and, if the force is too great, one or more of them will be damaged or torn. The most common position at the time of injury is a supinated foot combined with a plantarflexed ankle. The ligament damage occurs from anterior to posterior, with the anterior talofibular ligament being torn first. The mechanism of injury is an external perturbation that places the foot and ankle in the at risk position combined with a sudden high force. For example, landing from a jump partially on an opponent's foot in basketball or unexpectedly stepping off a high kerb while running. After the first ankle sprain, an athlete is at increased risk for spraining the ankle again. An athlete who experiences episodes of the ankle 'giving way' and typically suffers from multiple ankle sprains has chronic ankle instability. There are two main categories of chronic ankle instability: mechanical instability and functional instability. In mechanical ankle instability, the ligaments no longer restrain the ankle effectively – they may be elongated or even no longer intact and this allows the ankle to move into extreme positions. Alternatively, functional ankle instability is characterized by normal ligamentous restraint and instability is due to poor neuromuscular control. This may be attributed to loss of proprioception at the ankle leading to ineffective active muscular control of ankle position. Some athletes sprain their ankle and have no further symptoms – they are often referred to as 'copers' and there is a lot of research interest in understanding why and how they are able to cope with the injury. Athletes with chronic ankle instability often protect their ankle with rigid ankle braces that limit the amount of supination. Taping may also be used, but its effectiveness decreases with time as the tape loses adhesion to the skin due to sweating and limits prolonged activity. Rehabilitation programmes that aim to improve ankle proprioception and neuromuscular control may also help to reduce the risk of reinjury.

Further Reading

de Vries, J. S., Krips, R., Sierevelt, I. N., Blankevoort, L., & van Dijk, C. N. (2011). Interventions for treating chronic ankle instability. *Cochrane Database of Systematic Reviews*, 8. Art. No.: CD004124. DOI: 10.1002/14651858.CD004124.pub3.

Gribble, P. A., Bleakley, C. M., Caulfield, B. M., Docherty, C. L., Fourchet, F., Fong, D. T., ... Delahunt, E. (2016). Evidence review for the 2016 International Ankle Consortium consensus statement on the prevalence, impact and long-term consequences of lateral ankle sprains. *British Journal of Sports Medicine*, 50(24), 1496. DOI: 10.1136/bjsports-2016-096189.

Ankle and Foot – Bones

The ankle and foot contain many bones and joints, giving the region high mobility. As the first point of contact between the body and the ground, this flexible segment enables the individual to adapt easily to changes in terrain. The bones of the ankle joint are those of the distal part of the leg – the tibia and fibula – and the talus. The 26 bones of the foot are the talus, calcaneus, navicular, cuboid, and the 3 cuneiforms – these are the tarsal bones – plus the 5 metatarsal bones and the 14 phalanges (Figure 5).

The talus is common to both the ankle and the foot, forming the distal part of the ankle joint and the proximal part of the subtalar joint. The distal ends of the tibia and fibula, the malleoli, form the proximal part of the ankle joint and can be used to approximate the ankle joint axis *in vivo*. The ankle joint axis passes just distal to the tips of the malleoli. According to Inman (1976), the ankle joint axis lies, on average, 5 mm distal to the tip of the medial malleolus, and 3 mm distal and 8 mm anterior to the tip of the lateral malleolus.

The bones of the foot and ankle are at risk of stress fracture, particularly in runners and military recruits. Stress fractures commonly occur in the navicular, the metatarsals and the distal third of the tibia. There is some evidence that the incidence of these overuse injuries is higher in those individuals who have narrower tibiae, since these bones are less able to resist the bending forces to which the leg is subjected when the foot contacts the ground on every stride. Furthermore, stress fractures occur twice as often in females than in males, although the reasons for this difference are unclear. Owing to the seriousness of stress fractures, which require several weeks rest from training and physical activity until the bone is healed, they are an important research topic for sports biomechanists and physiotherapists. Factors that are thought to be related to the risk of stress fracture include structural anatomy, functional mechanics, footwear and training surface, training load, training frequency, and sex (see **Hot Topic 2**).

Reference

Inman, V. T. (1976). *The Joints of the Ankle*. Baltimore, MD: Williams & Wilkins.

Further Reading

Kelikian, A. S. (Ed.) (2011). *Sarrafian's anatomy of the foot and ankle: Descriptive, topographic, functional* (3rd ed.). Philadelphia, PA: Lippincott Williams & Wilkins.

See also: ankle and foot; ankle and foot – joints; ankle and foot – ligaments; ankle and foot – muscles; foot arches.

(a) Lateral view

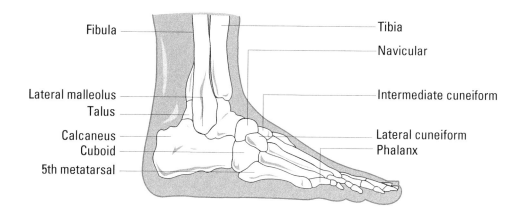

Fibula

Lateral malleolus
Talus
Calcaneus
Cuboid
5th metatarsal

Tibia
Navicular

Intermediate cuneiform

Lateral cuneiform
Phalanx

(b) Medial view

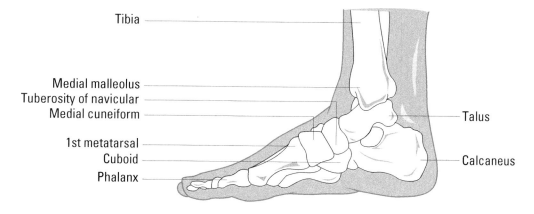

Tibia

Medial malleolus
Tuberosity of navicular
Medial cuneiform

1st metatarsal
Cuboid
Phalanx

Talus

Calcaneus

Figure 5 Bones of the right ankle and foot

Hot Topic 2 Barefoot Running

There has been an explosion of interest in barefoot running in the popular media in the past few years. Many anecdotal stories have touted it as a cure-all for running-related injuries. Others tell the opposite story. Only recently has an evidence base started to be built up around barefoot running in the biomechanics and sports medicine research literature. As sports and exercise scientists, it is essential to look to evidence in the peer-reviewed literature to evaluate whether barefoot running may be a good option for an individual runner. As with many prevention and treatment options for sports injuries, the evidence base is incomplete. One argument in support of barefoot running is that it is more 'natural' because ancient humans did not wear shoes. However, we should also take into account our modern habit of wearing shoes from our earliest steps, indicating that we are undoubtedly conditioned to wearing shoes. Of course, runners can choose to transition to running barefoot if it appeals to them. There is a risk of new injuries, particularly to the feet, if the transition to barefoot running is made too quickly. As with all changes in training stimulus, the tissues of the body need time to adapt to the new loads and load distributions and to remodel to be able to handle them. This is especially true the more novel the change.

Footwear manufacturers soon joined the barefoot running trend with at first 'barefoot shoes' and later 'minimal shoes'. A large body of literature is developing that encompasses barefoot running, minimal footwear, acute and chronic changes in running biomechanics, injury tracking and epidemiology, in attempts to tease out which aspects of barefoot running are critical in relation to injury. Key differences between shod and barefoot running that have been suggested to reduce injury risk include: adopting a forefoot strike pattern (landing on the front part of the foot first, not the heel), adopting a higher step rate (running cadence), strengthening the intrinsic muscles of the foot, and reducing impact loading. Of particular interest to runners and researchers is identifying minimal footwear that provides some protection to the foot from damage due to hazards on the running surface while mimicking any desirable features of barefoot running. Like all training and technique modifications designed to reduce the risk of injury, adopting barefoot running or wearing minimal shoes is not a one-size-fits-all approach.

Further Reading

Hall, J. P. L., Barton, C., Jones, P. R., & Morrissey, D. (2013). The biomechanical differences between barefoot and shod distance running: A systematic review and meta-analysis. *Sports Medicine, 43,* 1335–1353.

Ankle and Foot – Joints

The ankle and foot form a complex of many joints that provides flexibility and enables the foot to adapt to its environment. This flexibility of the foot is essential because it is the point of contact between the ground and the body; it must be able to adapt to changes in terrain with minimum perturbation of the body system as a whole. The foot is often divided into three sections based on its major articulations. The rear foot consists of the ankle and subtalar joints, the midfoot contains the calcaneocuboid, cuneonavicular, cuboideonavicular, intercuneiform, and cuneocuboid joints, and the forefoot consists of the tarsometatarsal, intermetatarsal, metatarsophalangeal, and interphalangeal joints. The greatest range of foot and ankle motion occurs at the rear foot.

The ankle, or talocrural, joint is the link between the leg and the foot. It approximates a hinge joint, with the talus of the foot being surrounded by the lateral malleolus, the medial malleolus and the distal end of the tibia. Sagittal plane flexion-extension movements at the ankle are known as plantarflexion, pointing the toes away from the leg, and dorsiflexion, pulling the toes towards the leg. From the neutral position, with the foot at 90° to the leg, the ankle can move into about 20° of dorsiflexion and 50° of plantarflexion.

The subtalar, or talocalcaneal, joint is formed between the distal surface of the talus and the proximal surface of the calcaneus. The subtalar joint axis is oriented obliquely in an anteromedial and superior direction. Since the joint axis is not aligned with any of the three cardinal planes of the body, movements about it are described as triplanar, with rotations occurring about all three anatomical axes. Movement about the subtalar joint axis is described as pronation, in which the rear foot rolls inwards towards its medial side, or supination, in which the rear foot rolls in the opposite direction. Rear foot pronation consists of eversion, dorsiflexion, and external rotation; its converse, supination, is made up of inversion, plantarflexion, and internal rotation.

The subtalar joint plays an important role in the shock absorption mechanism of the foot, owing to the changing properties of the foot as it moves from the rigid supinated position to the flexible pronated position. Abnormalities of rear foot motion have been associated with overuse injuries that can occur during running. During walking and running, the rotation of the rear foot about the subtalar joint axis helps to attenuate the forces transmitted through the foot and into the contact limb at foot strike. In a normal gait cycle, the foot contacts the ground in a supinated position, with the posterolateral part of the heel contacting first. The foot then moves into pronation, reaching a maximum towards the middle of the stance phase when the foot is flat on the ground. Finally, the foot returns to supination at toe off. The large rotation movement at foot strike, from supination to maximum pronation, is a shock-absorbing mechanism. The rate of pronation of the rear foot of the support limb at foot strike has been implicated in injury risk. Similarly, the maximum pronation reached during midstance is also thought to be linked to overuse injuries of the lower extremities, such as patellofemoral pain and Achilles tendon injury. The foot returns to supination towards toe off to provide a rigid lever during the push off at the end of stance phase. Failure of the foot to return to its rigid configuration has also been linked with overuse injury.

The joints of the midfoot have a much smaller range of motion than those of the rear foot and function mainly by gliding and rotating, providing a link between the independently articulating rear foot and forefoot regions.

The metatarsophalangeal joints at the base of the toes also play an important role during locomotion and have a large range of flexion-extension motion. Active extension in these joints, curling the toes up towards the ankle from the neutral position, is typically 50° to 60°, much greater than the 30° or 40° of flexion that can be achieved from that position; this is an adaptation to the role of the foot during walking. During toe off at the end of the stance phase of gait, the ankle is plantarflexed and the foot is supinated to provide a rigid lever to push off from the ground. The large extension possible at the metatarsophalangeal joints enables more of the toe region to remain in contact with the ground as the ankle plantarflexes and points the foot during this push off phase. This provides a larger base of support during the terminal stance phase.

Further Reading

Levine, D., Richards, J., & Whittle, M. W. (Eds.) (2012). *Whittle's gait analysis* (5th ed.), Oxford: Churchill Livingstone Elsevier.

See also: ankle and foot; ankle and foot – bones; ankle and foot – ligaments; ankle and foot – muscles.

Ankle and Foot – Ligaments

The ankle and foot contain many small bones and these are held together by ligaments (Figure 6). The ligaments of the ankle are grouped into lateral and medial collateral ligaments. The ankle ligaments are named according to the bones that they join together. Key bones are the leg bones – the tibia and fibula – which form the proximal part of the ankle joint, and the foot bones – the talus and the calcaneus. The lateral collateral ligament complex consists of the anterior talofibular ligament, the calcaneofibular ligament, and the posterior talofibular ligament. The three ligaments are thin bands of tissue and are relatively weak and susceptible to injury. The lateral ankle ligaments are the most commonly damaged ligaments in the body. The mechanism of injury is to 'roll' or 'sprain' your ankle, the common description of an inversion injury. When you sprain your ankle in this way, the anterior ligament is torn first, followed by the calcaneofibular and then the posterior ligament, as the severity of the injury increases. If the ligaments do not heal correctly, either remaining incomplete or becoming longer than before the injury, the ankle will be mechanically unstable and at greater risk of further injury to the lateral ligament. Following ligament damage, joint proprioception is typically reduced, which is also a factor in the predisposition of the individual for future recurrence of the injury (see **In Sports 1**).

The medial collateral ligament of the ankle is also known as the deltoid ligament because it is triangular in shape. The deltoid ligament is thick and strong and not divided into discrete bands like the lateral collateral ligaments. However, the medial ligaments of the ankle can also be identified according to the bones that they hold together. The names of the individual components vary slightly depending on which textbook you read, precisely because they are not conveniently separated like the lateral ligaments. The following is the common nomenclature for the components of the deltoid ligament. From anterior to posterior: tibionavicular (part of this ligament also attaches to the talus, referred to as anterior tibiotalar), tibiocalcaneal, and posterior tibiotalar. Since the deltoid ligament is thick and strong, it is not commonly injured. However, the mechanism of injury is the opposite movement to the mechanism of injury of the lateral collateral ligaments: an eversion sprain.

In addition to the medial and lateral collateral ligaments, there are two other ligaments at the distal end of the tibia and fibula. These are the anterior and posterior tibiofibular ligaments. These short ligaments bind the distal end of

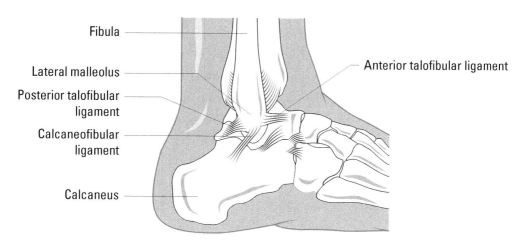

(a) Lateral view

Fibula

Lateral malleolus

Posterior talofibular ligament

Calcaneofibular ligament

Calcaneus

Anterior talofibular ligament

(b) Medial view

Medial malleolus

Anterior tibiotalar part of medial ligament of ankle

Navicular

Tibia

Talus

Posterior tibiotalar

Tibionavicular

Tibiocalcaneal

Parts of medial deltoid ligament of ankle

Calcaneus

Figure 6 Ligaments of the right ankle and foot

the tibia and fibular together tightly, to minimize any movement between them. The distal tibiofibular joint can effectively be considered to be immovable, with nothing more than a small amount of 'give' possible between the two leg bones.

There are many ligaments in the foot, too many to name individually. Their main function is to maintain the integrity of the foot system, which consists of 26 different bones. Since the foot has to function both as a flexible shock absorber during contact with the ground and a rigid lever while pushing off from the ground, the ligaments must allow some movement between adjacent bones, but not a large amount. The shape of the bones of the foot and the way that they fit together also provide a large amount of stability in the foot, as do the intrinsic and extrinsic foot muscles. Finally, another soft tissue structure, the plantar fascia (plantar aponeurosis), runs along the sole of the foot and provides additional support for the **foot arches**.

Further Reading

Kelikian, A. S. (Ed.) (2011). *Sarrafian's anatomy of the foot and ankle: Descriptive, topographic, functional* (3rd ed.). Philadelphia, PA: Lippincott Williams & Wilkins.

See also: ankle and foot; ankle and foot – bones; ankle and foot – joints; ankle and foot – muscles; foot arches.

Ankle and Foot – Muscles

The ankle and foot form a complex structure containing many bones and joints, which provide flexibility and enable the foot to adapt to its environment. This flexibility is essential because the foot is the first point of contact between the ground and the body and must be able to adapt to changes in terrain with minimum perturbation of the body as a whole. The muscles of the foot and ankle enable this flexible structure to perform different roles. For example, during walking and running, the foot acts as both a shock absorber and a rigid lever at different points in the gait cycle.

The muscles of the ankle and foot can be divided into four groups: the anterior leg muscles, the posterior leg (calf) muscles, the lateral leg muscles and the intrinsic muscles of the foot (Figure 7). The anterior muscles are the tibialis anterior, the

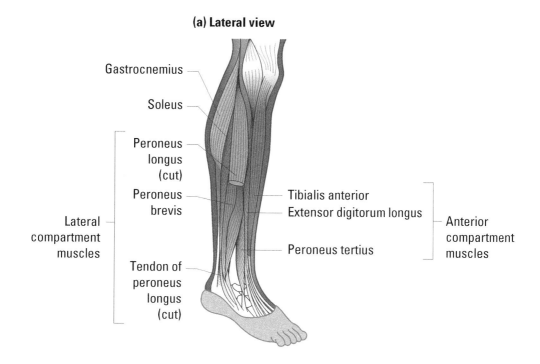

(a) Lateral view

Gastrocnemius

Soleus

Lateral compartment muscles

Peroneus longus (cut)

Peroneus brevis

Tendon of peroneus longus (cut)

Tibialis anterior

Extensor digitorum longus

Peroneus tertius

Anterior compartment muscles

(b) Anterior view

Soleus

Peroneus longus

Gastrocnemius

Soleus

Anterior compartment muscles

Tibialis anterior

Extensor digitorum longus

Extensor hallucis longus

Peroneus tertius

Figure 7 Muscles of the right ankle and foot. Adapted from Sewell et al. (2013).

Table 1 Ankle and foot muscles contributing to joint movements

Joint movement	Muscles
Ankle dorsiflexion	Tibialis anterior, peroneus tertius, extensor digitorum longus, extensor hallucis longus
Ankle plantarflexion	Gastrocnemius, soleus, tibialis posterior, peroneus longus, peroneus brevis, flexor digitorum longus, flexor hallucis longus, plantaris
Rearfoot supination	Tibialis anterior, tibialis posterior, flexor digitorum longus
Rearfoot pronation	Peroneus longus, peroneus brevis, peroneus tertius
Toe extension	Extensor digitorum longus, extensor hallucis longus
Toe flexion	Flexor digitorum longus, flexor hallucis longus

Pronation consists of eversion, dorsiflexion and external rotation. Supination consists of inversion, plantarflexion and internal rotation.

peroneus tertius, the extensor digitorum longus, and the extensor hallucis longus. As a group, these muscles cross the front of the ankle and dorsiflex the ankle. In addition, the tibialis anterior supinates the foot, the peroneus tertius pronates the foot, the extensor digitorum longus extends the four lesser toes and pronates the foot, and the extensor hallucis longus supinates the foot and extends the big toe (Table 1).

The posterior muscles of the ankle and foot are gastrocnemius, soleus, plantaris, flexor digitorum longus, flexor hallucis longus, and tibialis posterior. As a group, these muscles cross the back of the ankle and plantarflex the ankle. Gastrocnemius is the large two-headed muscle that forms the bulk of the calf and also flexes the knee (see **knee – muscles**) and supinates the foot. The next largest muscle of the calf is soleus, which lies deep to the gastrocnemius; its action is purely plantarflexing the ankle. Between these two muscles lies the small plantaris muscle, which makes a minor contribution to flexing the knee and plantarflexing the ankle. Deep to these muscles lies popliteus; this muscle contributes to flexing the knee and internally rotating the tibia. Flexors digitorum and hallucis longus flex the four lesser toes and great toe respectively. Tibialis posterior supinates the foot in addition to plantarflexing the ankle. Two muscles are situated laterally on the leg, peroneus longus and peroneus brevis. Their role is pronating the foot and plantarflexing the ankle. The intrinsic muscles of the foot contribute to movement of the toes. There are many muscles within the foot, with the muscles of the dorsum of the foot being four layers deep.

Further Reading

Kelikian, A. S. (Ed.) (2011). *Sarrafian's anatomy of the foot and ankle: Descriptive, topographic, functional* (3rd ed.). Philadelphia, PA: Lippincott Williams & Wilkins.

See also: ankle and foot; ankle and foot – bones; ankle and foot – joints; ankle and foot – ligaments; foot arches.

Elbow and Forearm

The elbow joint complex consists of a hinge joint between the humerus of the arm and the ulna of the forearm plus a secondary hinge joint between the radius of the forearm and the humerus, both of which are constrained to uniaxial flexion-extension motion (see **planes and axes of movement**). A third joint occurs between the bones of the forearm: the proximal radioulnar joint, which is often considered to be part of the elbow joint because it is contained within the same articular capsule. The radioulnar joint allows pronation-supination of the forearm, which enables the hand to assume a pronated or supinated position at any elbow flexion angle.

In sports that have a large involvement of the upper extremity, the elbow is at risk of overuse injury. Large forces can be transmitted across the joint in hitting sports such as tennis and baseball. Overuse injuries can range from the severity of ligament tears to tissue inflammation at tendon insertions caused by overuse of the muscle involved. These injuries may be related to incorrect technique or simple overload. The many degrees of freedom of the upper extremity mean that a given movement of the hand can be achieved by many different positions and orientations of the proximal segments of the limb. Poor technique overstresses certain tissues and, as a result of the repetition of practice and competition, relatively minor deviations from the correct structural alignment of the limb can result in cumulative damage leading to overuse injury.

See also: **appendicular skeleton; elbow and forearm – bones; elbow and forearm – joints; elbow and forearm – ligaments; elbow and forearm – muscles.**

Elbow and Forearm – Bones

The ulnohumeral joint is a hinge joint between the trochlea of the humerus in the arm and the trochlear notch of the ulna in the forearm of the upper extremity; its motion is sagittal plane flexion-extension (see **planes and axes of movement**). The entire joint comprises three articulations between the three long bones of the upper limb (Figure 8). These are the ulnohumeral joint already described, the radiohumeral joint between the head of the radius of the forearm and the capitulum of the humerus, and the proximal radiohumeral joint. The head of the radius is constrained by the anular ligament at the proximal radioulnar

(a) Anterior view

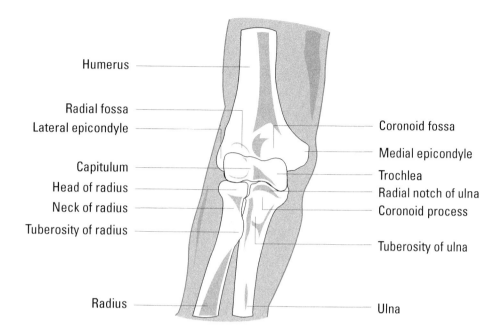

Humerus

Radial fossa

Lateral epicondyle

Capitulum

Head of radius

Neck of radius

Tuberosity of radius

Radius

Coronoid fossa

Medial epicondyle

Trochlea

Radial notch of ulna

Coronoid process

Tuberosity of ulna

Ulna

(b) Posterior view

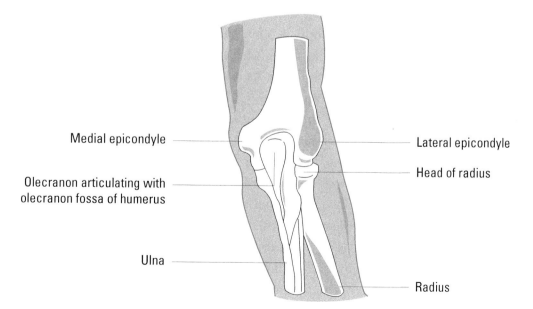

Medial epicondyle

Olecranon articulating with
olecranon fossa of humerus

Ulna

Lateral epicondyle

Head of radius

Radius

Figure 8 Bones of the right elbow and forearm

joint. This joint enables pronation and supination of the forearm by rotation of the radius within the anular ligament. Stabilization of the elbow is provided by both the bony structure of the ulnohumeral joint, with the trochlear sitting in the trochlear notch, and by the soft tissues. Important soft tissue stabilizers are the joint capsule, the medial and lateral collateral ligaments, and the anular ligament.

Traumatic injuries to the forearm are relatively common in team sports such as soccer. A player may fall and land awkwardly with the arm extended to cushion the impact of the fall. Such a fall can result in fracture of the forearm or dislocation of the shoulder joint (see **shoulder complex – joints**).

See also: **elbow and forearm; elbow and forearm – joints; elbow and forearm – ligaments; elbow and forearm – muscles.**

Elbow and Forearm – Joints

The elbow consists of three joints all within the same joint capsule. The major articulation of the elbow is the hinge joint between the humerus of the upper arm and the ulna of the forearm. This ulnohumeral joint is responsible for flexion-extension of the elbow joint. Mediolateral movement at the joint is prevented by its bony structure (see **planes and axes of movement**). The distal end of the humerus, the trochlea, sits in the trochlear notch at the proximal end of the ulna. The second joint at the elbow is between the radius of the forearm and the humerus. This radiohumeral joint is not constrained by its bony structure. It is the articulation between the capitulum and the head of the radius. The radiohumeral joint would be susceptible to dislocation if the thick annular ligament, which forms a ring around the proximal end of the radius, was not present to stabilize it. The third joint at the elbow, the proximal radioulnar joint, between the radial head and the ulnar notch, enables pronation-supination of the forearm and, therefore, repositions the hand about the long axis of the upper limb.

The elbow commonly suffers from overuse injury, particularly in racquet or other hitting sports. The classic overuse injury of the elbow is lateral epicondylitis, also known as 'tennis elbow'. The injury is characterized by inflammation or degeneration of the tissues at the insertion of the wrist extensor tendons at the lateral epicondyle. Its occurrence is often linked to technical faults that result in excessive tension and stretch in the forearm muscles of the playing arm. A common backhand fault is using excessive wrist extension in an attempt to give more power to the shot. Using a double-handed backhand avoids this technique and emphasizes power from the trunk and shoulder. In addition to technique faults, equipment can also contribute to excessive loading of the extensor muscles of the forearm. Heavy or large racquets, particularly those with most of their weight in the head, increase the load on the muscles of the forearm in maintaining racquet position. A racquet with highly-tensioned strings will result in more force being transmitted up the arm, rather than dissipating some of the contact force in the racquet itself.

Further Reading

Dines, J. S., Bedi, A., Williams, P. N., Dodson, C. C., Ellenbecker, T. S., Altchek, D. W., . . . Dines, D. M. (2015). Tennis injuries: Epidemiology, pathophysiology, and treatment. *Journal of the American Academy of Orthopedic Surgeons, 23*, 181–189.

See also: elbow and forearm; elbow and forearm – bones; elbow and forearm – joints; elbow and forearm – ligaments; elbow and forearm – muscles.

Elbow and Forearm – Ligaments

The elbow joint includes the ulnohumeral, radiohumeral and proximal radioulnar joints. This complex joint is held together by several extracapsular ligaments (Figure 9). On the sides of the joint are the medial and lateral collateral ligaments, which are also referred to as the ulnar and radial collateral ligaments. The medial collateral ligament runs from the medial humeral epicondyle to the coronoid process and olecranon of the ulna. The lateral collateral ligament runs from the lateral epicondyle of the humerus to the anular ligament. These two ligaments check movement of the ulnohumeral and radiohumeral joints in flexion and extension, as well as checking the small amount of abduction and adduction which occurs at the elbow.

The forearm is a unique structure because the two bones within it, the ulna and radius, are able to move from their normal side-by-side position to a crossed position. This movement is pronation-supination and is possible because of a special ligamentous structure around the head of the radius. The anular ligament

(a) Medial view

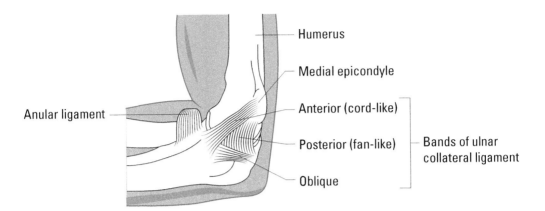

(b) Lateral view

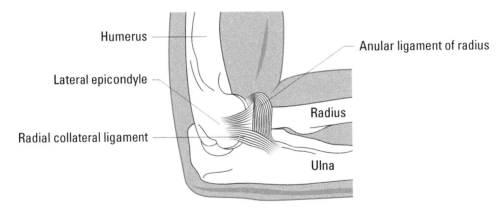

Figure 9 Ligaments of the right elbow and forearm

is a ring of tissue which surrounds the head of the radius at the proximal end of the forearm. The proximal radioulnar joint is a pivot joint, meaning that the radius rotates about its long axis as the head rotates within the anular ligament. This movement, along with pivoting at the distal radioulnar joint, results in the radius crossing over the ulna as the forearm moves into pronation. There is an additional structure, the interosseous membrane, which provides further support to the bones of the forearm. The interosseous membrane runs the length of the shaft of the forearm bones, filling in the space between them.

See also: **elbow and forearm; elbow and forearm – bones; elbow and forearm – joints; elbow and forearm – muscles.**

Elbow and Forearm – Muscles

The muscles of the elbow and forearm can be divided into five groups: the muscles of the arm that are involved with movements at the elbow joint, and four groups in the forearm (Figure 10; Table 2). The forearm muscles are divided into anterior and posterior groups, and then subdivided further into superficial and deep groups. The muscles of the arm that cross the front of the elbow and are responsible for flexing it are: biceps brachii, the large muscle on the front of the arm; brachialis which is deep to biceps brachii; and brachioradialis, a smaller muscle that inserts into the base of the radial styloid process. The biceps also contributes to supinating the forearm and stabilizing the shoulder joint. The biceps also crosses the front of the shoulder and is a weak shoulder flexor. The muscles arising from the medial epicondyle of the humerus are the superficial flexors of the forearm that flex the wrist and can also contribute to flexing the elbow. The extensors of the elbow cross the back of the joint and are the triceps brachii on the back of the humerus and the small anconeus.

The superficial muscles on the anterior aspect of the forearm are the pronator teres, flexor carpi radialis, palmaris longus, flexor carpi ulnaris, and flexor digitorum superficialis, all of which originate from the medial humeral epicondyle at the elbow. These muscles act variously in pronating the forearm and flexing, abducting, and adducting the wrist (see **wrist and hand – muscles**). The deep anterior muscles of the forearm are the flexor digitorum profundus and flexor pollicis longus, which flex the fingers and thumb respectively. Additionally, pronator quadratus is a deep anterior muscle that pronates the forearm.

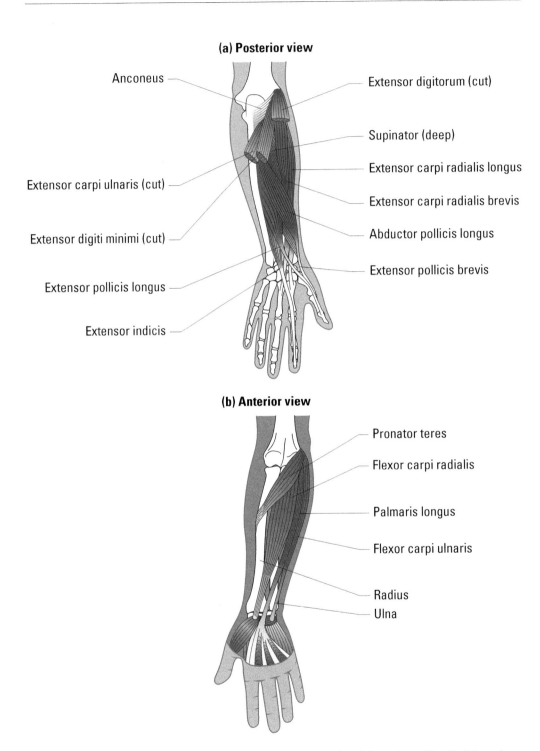

(a) Posterior view

Anconeus

Extensor digitorum (cut)

Supinator (deep)

Extensor carpi radialis longus

Extensor carpi ulnaris (cut)

Extensor carpi radialis brevis

Extensor digiti minimi (cut)

Abductor pollicis longus

Extensor pollicis longus

Extensor pollicis brevis

Extensor indicis

(b) Anterior view

Pronator teres

Flexor carpi radialis

Palmaris longus

Flexor carpi ulnaris

Radius

Ulna

Figure 10 Muscles of the right elbow and forearm (including muscles of the wrist and hand). Adapted from Sewell et al. (2013).

Table 2 Elbow and forearm muscles contributing to joint movements

Joint movement	Muscles
Elbow flexion	Biceps brachii, brachialis, brachioradialis, prontator teres
Elbow extension	Triceps brachii, anconeus
Forearm supination	Biceps brachii, supinator
Forearm pronation	Pronator teres, pronator quadratus

See Table 9 for forearm muscles contributing to wrist joint movements.

The superficial muscles on the posterior aspect of the forearm originate on the lateral epicondyle. They are extensor carpi radialis longus, extensor carpi radialis brevis, extensor digitorum, extensor digiti minimi, and extensor carpi ulnaris. These muscles extend, abduct and adduct the wrist, and extend the digits (see **wrist and hand – muscles**). The deep muscles of the posterior forearm are: supinator, which supinates the forearm; abductor pollicis longus, extensor pollicis brevis, extensor pollicis longus, which extend and abduct the thumb; and extensor indicis, which extends the index finger.

The muscles of the elbow and forearm are at risk of both traumatic and overuse injury. Traumatic ruptures of the tendon of either biceps or triceps brachii are relatively uncommon, but may occur when large forces are exerted quickly on the tendon. An athlete will usually be able to recall a specific moment when the injury occurred. This injury is serious and requires surgical repair to give an athlete the best chance of regaining their pre-injury ability. Overuse injuries in this region are typically epicondylitis at the elbow, inflammation of the tendon attachments. Common examples are tennis elbow, or lateral epicondylitis (see **elbow and forearm – joints; In Sports 2**), and golfer's elbow, or medial epicondylitis. These injuries are often due to errors in technique, making them particularly common in novice players.

See also: **elbow and forearm; elbow and forearm – bones; elbow and forearm – joints; elbow and forearm – ligaments.**

In Sports 2 Tennis Elbow

Tennis elbow is an overuse injury of the wrist extensor muscles which causes irritation at the lateral epicondyle of the elbow. This injury, formally known as 'lateral epicondylitis' is common in tennis players due to the repeated wrist extension action during tennis strokes. While the joint movement is at the wrist, the pain associated with the injury is felt at the elbow. The lateral epicondyle of the elbow is the common origin for the long wrist extensor muscles and is subjected to high tensile strains when the extensor muscles repeatedly generate high forces. Tennis elbow is more common in novice or recreational tennis players than elite players and it is attributed to faulty technique. Studies of muscle activity have shown that the wrist extensor muscles are more active in players with tennis elbow compared to those without the injury. High loads are transmitted through the arm and forearm during the tennis stroke, particularly during impact with the ball. Faulty stroke biomechanics associated with wrist extension and high demand on the wrist extensor muscles put the player at risk for injury. Overuse injuries develop due to a combination of high repetitions and high loads. High repetition of strokes during practice and matches leads to an accumulation of damage and the onset of pain associated with the injury. As with all overuse injuries, recovery typically starts with refraining from the aggravating activity and substituting other conditioning activities until the pain subsides. A padded brace placed on the upper forearm may help to reduce the load on the epicondyle during everyday activities. When the injury can be attributed to a technique fault related to incorrect biomechanics, technique modification is an important part of the rehabilitation process. In the case of tennis elbow, switching from a one-handed to a two-handed backhand is often recommended to reduce the load on the wrist extensors during the stroke.

Further Reading

De Smedt, T., de Jong, A., Van Leemput, W., Lieven, D., & Van Glabbeek, F. (2007). Lateral epicondylitis in tennis: Update on aetiology, biomechanics and treatment. *British Journal of Sports Medicine, 41*(11), 816. doi: 10.1136/bjsm.2007.036723.

Foot Arches

The foot has three arches: the medial longitudinal arch, the shorter lateral longitudinal arch, and the transverse arch. These arches enable the foot to safely and effectively transmit large loads during contact with the ground. The bony structure of the foot and its soft tissues both contribute to the integrity of the foot arches. The plantar fascia, also known as the plantar aponeurosis, is the key soft tissue structure associated with the foot arches. This strong and wide band runs under the sole of the foot from the heel to the toes. Its connection to both the rear foot and forefoot helps to prevent the bony structure of the foot from collapsing when a downward vertical load is applied to it, as during weight bearing. Lack of appropriate soft tissue support causes the foot to be excessively flexible, reducing its effectiveness as a rigid lever when pushing off from the ground. This is commonly known as 'flat feet' or pes planus.

A common overuse injury associated with the arches of the feet is plantar fasciitis, caused by repetitive overload of the plantar fascia. The symptoms are pain under the heel of the foot that is worse early in the morning and after excessive standing. This injury may be resolved by providing support for the plantar fascia by use of orthotics (see **Hot Topic 3**) or by strengthening the intrinsic foot muscles, both of which aim to lessen the tensile load on the fascia.

See also: ankle and foot; ankle and foot – bones; ankle and foot – joints; ankle and foot – ligaments; ankle and foot – muscles.

Hot Topic 3 Foot Orthotic Devices

In-shoe foot orthotics are often prescribed to prevent recurrent overuse injuries in runners and other athletes. The purpose of a foot orthotic is to provide support for the foot and keep it in good alignment as weight is transferred onto the foot during walking, running, and other weight-bearing activities. In many cases, orthotics are intended to provide support in the region of the medial longitudinal arch of a flat foot (see **foot arches**). Plantar fasciitis is a painful foot injury in which the insertion of the plantar fascia on the calcaneus (heel bone) becomes inflamed due to excessive loading of the plantar fascia. The plantar fascia is a key support structure for the medial longitudinal arch of the foot and is placed under tension when the foot pronates excessively and the arch collapses. The use of an orthotic can provide support for the arch and prevent this extreme position from being reached. This reduces the irritation of the insertion of the plantar fascia and may prevent the injury from recurring.

The research literature related to the effectiveness of orthotics in the treatment of pain and prevention of injury is inconclusive. However, many people have great success in resolving their pain with orthotics. Part of the reason for the conflicting reports may be that there are so many types of orthotic available. Mass-produced off the shelf orthotics can be purchased cheaply, but may not suit the individual foot type or provide support in the right places. Orthotics can be custom-made for the individual by a podiatrist or physiotherapist. In this case, the clinician makes a cast of the foot and then decides how much to reposition the foot, how much support to add and whether to use flexible or rigid materials. Due to the custom nature of this type of orthotic, the cost is much higher.

Further Reading

Bonanno, D. R., Landorf, K. B., Munteanu, S. E., Murley, G. S., & Menz, H. B. (2017). Effectiveness of foot orthoses and shock-absorbing insoles for the prevention of injury: A systematic review and meta-analysis. *British Journal of Sports Medicine, 51,* 86–96.

Head and Neck

The bones of the head and neck are those of the skull plus the seven cervical vertebrae. Most of the 22 bones of the skull are fused and form a strong protective case for the delicate tissues of the brain. The cervical vertebrae enable the neck to move in all three cardinal planes (see **planes and axes of movement**).

The skull is mainly at risk of traumatic injury owing to accidental contact with an opponent, sports equipment, or the ground. For example, if two players try to head the ball in a soccer match, they may accidentally hit each other and cause an injury, such as a broken nose. Similarly, in squash, contact with the opponent's racquet or the ball can lead to eye injuries. The neck and cervical spine are at risk of overuse injuries if extremes of head position are held for long periods. For example, cyclists may suffer from neck pain as a result of hyper-extending the neck to lift the head sufficiently to see ahead.

See also: **axial skeleton; head and neck – bones; head and neck – joints; head and neck – ligaments; head and neck – muscles.**

Head and Neck – Bones

The bones of the head and neck comprise the bones of the skull and the seven vertebrae of the cervical spine. The bones of the skull, which are fused in the adult, are the cranium – the large dome that houses and protects the brain – and the bones of the face (Figure 11). The skull is made up of 8 cranial and 14 facial bones. All of these, except the mandible (jawbone), are attached rigidly to each other by interlaced articulations called sutures. The bones of the skull are not fully fused at the sutures until old age and do not begin to close until about age 22 years, with the process being mostly complete by age 30. This should be taken into consideration when younger athletes suffer a traumatic injury to the head, since the skull serves to protect the delicate tissues of the brain. Damage to the bones of the skull tends to be due to acute trauma from contact with another athlete, equipment, or the ground.

The cranial bones are the occipital bone at the back of the head, the two parietal bones forming the sides and top of the cranium, the frontal bone of the forehead, the two temporal bones at the sides below the parietal bones in the region of the ears, the sphenoid bone at the base of the skull extending laterally in front of the

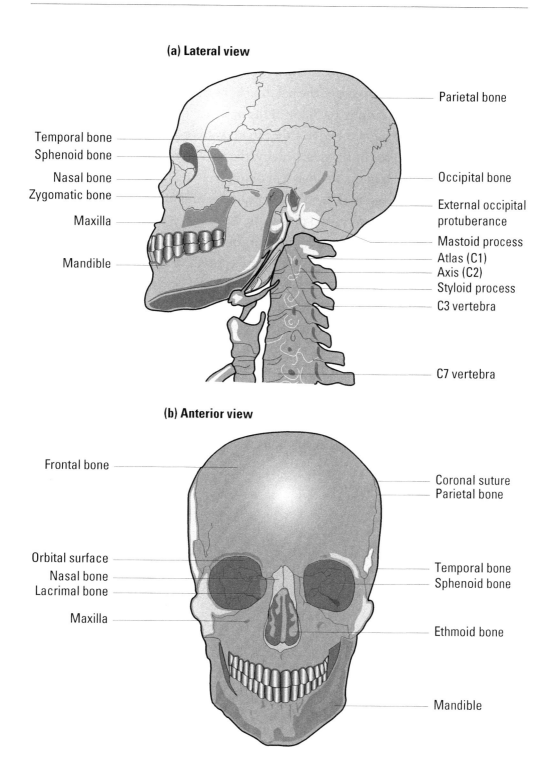

(a) Lateral view

Parietal bone

Temporal bone
Sphenoid bone
Nasal bone
Zygomatic bone
Maxilla

Mandible

Occipital bone

External occipital
protuberance

Mastoid process
Atlas (C1)
Axis (C2)
Styloid process
C3 vertebra

C7 vertebra

(b) Anterior view

Frontal bone

Coronal suture
Parietal bone

Orbital surface
Nasal bone
Lacrimal bone

Maxilla

Temporal bone
Sphenoid bone

Ethmoid bone

Mandible

Figure 11 Bones of the head and neck

temporal bones, and the ethmoid bone that forms the walls of the superior part of the nasal cavity. The facial bones are the two nasal bones – the bridge of the nose, the two maxillae of the upper jaw, the palatine bone behind the maxillae – forming parts of the roof of the mouth, the floor of the nasal cavity, and the floor of the eye orbit, the two inferior nasal conchae – the lateral walls of the nasal cavity, the two vomers that are also part of the nasal cavity, the two lacrimal bones – part of the eye orbit, and the two zygomatic (cheek) bones.

Injuries to the head and neck tend to be traumatic and often occur as a result of unintentional contact between two players in team sports such as soccer. Typical injuries include nosebleeds, broken noses, concussion (see **In Sports 3**), and fracture of the facial bones, and may be severe enough to require hospitalization. In some sports, such as cycling, protective headgear can be worn to reduce the risk of severe head trauma in the case of unintentional contact with the ground.

Racket sports are the most common source of sports-related eye injuries. Such injuries are caused by the racket, shuttlecock, or ball. The best protection from these injuries is to wear eye guards that prevent objects from entering the eye from any angle.

See also: **bone; bone classification; head and neck; head and neck – joints; head and neck – ligaments; head and neck – muscles; vertebral structure.**

In Sports 3 Concussion

Sports-related concussion has received a lot of attention in the media recently. Sports-related concussion is a mild traumatic brain injury caused by high velocity impact with a person or object. Rapid head accelerations resulting from the impact cause the brain to be jostled inside the cranial cavity of the skull, damaging the delicate tissue. Symptoms include dizziness and headaches, excessive tiredness, difficulty concentrating on a task, and visual disturbances. Common causes of sports-related concussion include player-to-player impact in American football, ice hockey, or soccer, receiving blows to the head in boxing or other contact martial arts, or head impact with the ball in soccer. Falls resulting in head contact with the ground are another cause of concussion in sports. Given the high risk of neurological damage in both the short and long term, reducing the risk of concussion in sports is important in protecting the safety of athletes. Rule changes and the use of protective equipment can help to reduce the incidence or severity of head impacts. For example, 'spearing' or leading with the head in a tackle is forbidden in American football. This rule was implemented in efforts to reduce the number and severity of head and neck injuries during player contact. In youth soccer in the United States limits have been set on the minimum age of players who are allowed to head the ball and limits on heading in youth players. Research tools such as instrumented helmets have been developed in efforts to quantify the magnitude and frequency of head accelerations associated with impact with other players or the ground during gameplay and practice in American football and other helmeted sports. New sideline screening tools to better evaluate players are also being developed to inform return-to-play decisions during a game.

Further Reading

Emery, C. A., Black, A. M., Kolstad, A., Martinez, G., Nettel-Aguirre, A., Engebretsen, L., ... Schneider, K. (2017). What strategies can be used to effectively reduce the risk of concussion in sport? A systematic review. *British Journal of Sports Medicine, 51*(12), 978. doi: 10.1136/bjsports-2016-097452.

O'Connor, K. L., Rowson, S., Duma, S. M., & Broglio, S. (2017). Head-impact-measurement devices: A systematic review. *Journal of Athletic Training, 52*(3), 206–227. doi: 10.4085/1062-6050.52.2.05.

Head and Neck – Joints

Most bones of the head are rigidly attached to each other by interwoven articulations known as sutures. The only moveable bone of the head is the mandible, or jawbone, which articulates with the temporal bones of the skull. The neck, containing the cervical spine, articulates with the cranium as well as adjacent vertebrae. The cervical spine carries the head and enables it to assume many different positions as a result of flexion-extension, axial rotation, and lateral flexion of the neck.

The two temporomandibular joints between the temporal bones of the skull and the jawbone are combined hinge and gliding joints. These joints enable the jaw to be opened and closed, protruded forward, and displaced laterally. In contact sports, such as boxing, the jaw is at risk of being broken or dislocated as a result of a direct blow to the face. This type of injury may also occur in contact team sports such as rugby.

The occipital bone of the skull rests on top of the first cervical vertebra, the atlas. The movements between these two bones are mainly flexion-extension; there is also a slight lateral motion of the head. Axial rotation of the atlas and, therefore, the skull, occurs at the joint between it and the axis – the second cervical vertebra. The joints between the individual vertebrae allow only a slight range of motion, but when the total for a region of the spine is added together, the range of motion is significant. The movements that can occur in the vertebral column are flexion-extension, lateral flexion, axial rotation, and circumduction. The largest range of motion is in flexion. All of these movements are greatest in the cervical spine, which is the most flexible part of the spinal column.

Overuse injuries to the joints can occur in the cervical region. Cyclists commonly suffer from such overuse injury. Neck pain can occur as a result of excessive hyperextension of the neck during cycling and typically affects the first three cervical vertebrae. The risk of overuse injury of the neck can be minimized by setting up the bicycle appropriately for the individual. Riding with the hands set too low in relation to the body, either by having the handlebars too low or spending too much time on the dropped part of the handlebar can contribute to this injury. Additionally, riding a bicycle that is too long and causes the rider to overreach will also put the rider in a disadvantageous position. Generally, raising the torso by attending to either of these set-up faults will resolve the neck pain.

General poor posture, in either everyday life or specific sports, can lead to neck pain. The cervical spine tends to be overloaded when other parts of the body are in poor alignment, because it is flexible and directly responsible for the position of the head.

See also: **head and neck; head and neck – bones; head and neck – ligaments; head and neck – muscles.**

Head and Neck – Ligaments

The majority of bones in the head are fused to each other via sutures to provide a protective shell for the brain. Movement occurs at the temporomandibular joint, to allow opening and closing of the mouth. There are several ligaments associated with this joint. The joint capsule is thickened into a lateral ligament, sometimes referred to as the temporomandibular ligament. This ligament adds support to the lateral aspect of the joint and helps to prevent posterior dislocation. There are two additional ligaments extrinsic to the temporomandibular joint: the stylomandibular and sphenomandibular ligaments. These ligaments connect the mandible to points on the cranium. The stylomandibular ligament runs from the styloid process of the temporal cranial bone to the angle of the mandible distally. The sphenomandibular ligament runs from the spine of the sphenoid cranial bone to the lingula of the mandible, which is superior to the insertion of the stylomandibular ligament.

The neck is the most proximal part of the vertebral column, the cervical region. Therefore, it has several ligaments in common with the thoracic and lumbar regions of the spine. These common ligaments are: the anterior and posterior longitudinal ligaments, ligamentum flavum, interspinous and supraspinous ligaments (see **thoracic region – ligaments**). There is an additional ligament unique to the cervical region: the nuchal ligament. This ligament runs medially on the posterior aspect of the neck. Specifically, it runs from the external occipital protuberance and posterior border of the foramen magnum of the skull to the spinous processes of the cervical vertebrae. The spinous processes are short in the cervical region of the vertebral column, so the strong and thick nuchal ligament provides a substitute for muscular attachment in this region.

See also: **head and neck; head and neck – bones; head and neck – joints; head and neck – muscles.**

Head and Neck – Muscles

Most muscles of the head and neck are involved in either facial expression or mastication (chewing) and are not directly involved in sports injuries, other than superficial bruising and contusions. The muscles of the neck, however, are heavily involved in sports activities because they are responsible for orienting the head via movements of the cervical spine (Table 3).

The lateral muscles of the neck are the trapezius and the sternocleidomastoid. Similar to the muscles on either side of the lumbar spine (see **lumbar spine and pelvis – muscles**), the action of the sternocleidomastoid muscles depends on whether one or both of them are active. Contraction of the muscle on one side of the head bends the neck laterally to the same side or rotates the head towards the opposite side. The action of both muscles together flexes the neck forwards. The trapezius is a large muscle that acts at the shoulder as well as the neck (see **shoulder complex – muscles**). Its role at the neck is to laterally flex the neck towards the side that is contracting, while rotating the head away from that side; trapezius extends the neck if both sides contract simultaneously.

Deep muscles attached directly to the vertebral column are also responsible for movements of the neck. Anteriorly on the neck, longus colli, longus capitis, and anterior rectus capitis contribute to forward flexion, and lateral rectus capitis flexes the neck laterally towards the side that is contracting. Posteriorly, the deep muscles of the back are responsible for extending the vertebral column. At the cervical level, the deep muscles responsible for extending and rotating the neck are

Table 3 Head and neck muscles contributing to joint movements

Joint movement	Muscles
Neck flexion	Both*: Sternocleidomastoid, longus colli, longus capitis, anterior rectus capitis
Neck extension	Both*: Trapezius, splenius, iliocostalis cervicis, longissimus capitis, spinalis capitis, semispinalis capitis
Neck lateral flexion to the right**	Right sternocleidomastoid, right trapezius, right splenius
Neck rotation to the right**	Left sternocleidomastoid, right splenius

Notes: * Both indicates this is the action when both muscles contract together.

** A direction is given for lateral flexion and rotation to illustrate whether the individual muscle on the same or opposite side to the direction of movement is active.

splenius, iliocostalis cervicis, longissimus capitis, spinalis capitis, and semispinalis capitis (see Figure 24).

The neck can be subject to both overuse and traumatic injury. Sports that require the neck to be held in the same extreme position for extended periods are prone to overuse injury as a result of the excess loading placed on the muscles involved. Examples of such injuries can be found in cycling, where the neck may be hyperextended to enable the eyes to look directly forwards (see **head and neck – joints**).

Strengthening the neck may protect it from traumatic injury caused by movements at the extremes of its range of motion. This type of injury is a particular risk in contact sports, such as wrestling and rugby, in which the neck may be in close contact with either an opponent or the ground. Neck strength can be increased by various means. For example, harnesses with weights attached can be worn hanging from the head to provide extra resistance for flexion and extension movements. These isolation exercises work specifically on neck strength but may not replicate very closely what happens during the sports activity. Various bridging exercises, in which athletes lie supine and then raise themselves up on to the top of the head and the soles of the feet while arching the back – followed by lowering the body under control – also strengthen the neck. The advantage of these exercises is that they also recruit the smaller stabilizing muscles of the head and neck region and improve both strength and awareness of body position that are vital to minimizing the risk of injury in sports.

See also: **head and neck; head and neck – bones; head and neck – joints; head and neck – ligaments.**

Hip

The hip joint is formed between the acetabulum of the hip bone in the pelvis, and the proximal end of the femur. The hip is the most mobile joint of the lower extremity and is able to rotate about all three axes (see **planes and axes of movement**) owing to its configuration as a ball and socket joint (see **joints**). The hip is a stable joint with many strong ligamentous attachments that contribute to its stability, in addition to its bony structure. As a result, it is dislocated much less frequently than its upper extremity equivalent, the glenohumeral (shoulder) joint (see **shoulder complex – joints**).

However, as a result of its structure and large ranges of motion in all three cardinal planes, the hip is implicated in overuse injuries of the lower extremities. For example, some runners run with the hip joint excessively internally rotated. Although the hip joint is easily able to accommodate this, rotation at the joint changes the alignment of the whole lower extremity, the distal joints of which are less able to adapt to the change. This places bony and soft tissue structures under increased loads as they try to accommodate the alignment at the hip alongside the constraints of foot contact with the ground during the gait cycle. Over the many repetitions of many miles of running during training and competition, this malalignment increases wear and tear on the tissues of the lower extremity and may lead to overuse injury. Despite the movement changes being at the hip, injury often occurs more distally in the lower extremity, at the knee.

See also: **hip – bones; hip – joint; hip – ligaments; hip – muscles.**

Hip – Bones

The hip is the most proximal joint of the lower extremity and has the greatest multiaxial range of motion of all the lower extremity joints. It is formed between the hip bone, which is part of the pelvis and consists of the ilium, ischium and pubis, and the femur, the long bone between the hip and the knee (Figure 12). The hip is a ball and socket joint (see **joints**) and, as such, makes the thigh and lower limb very mobile with respect to the pelvis. Because of its bony configuration, the joint is stabilized by both the cup-like acetabulum of the hip bone and the strong ligamentous attachments between it and the femur.

(a) Anterior view

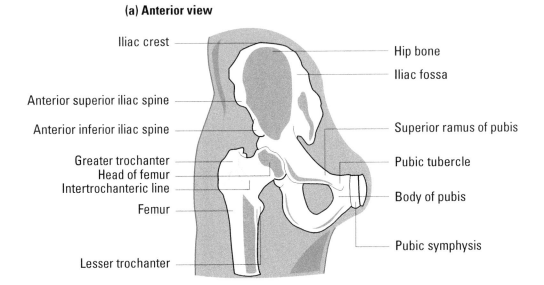

Iliac crest

Anterior superior iliac spine

Anterior inferior iliac spine

Greater trochanter
Head of femur
Intertrochanteric line
Femur

Lesser trochanter

Hip bone
Iliac fossa

Superior ramus of pubis

Pubic tubercle

Body of pubis

Pubic symphysis

(b) Posterior view

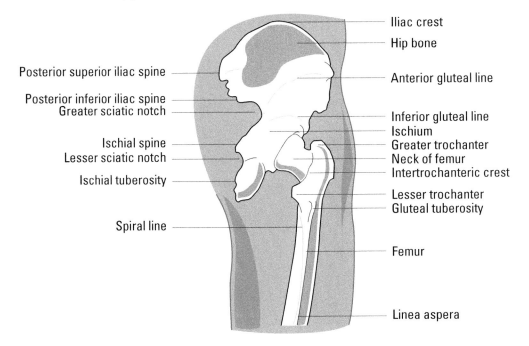

Posterior superior iliac spine

Posterior inferior iliac spine
Greater sciatic notch

Ischial spine
Lesser sciatic notch

Ischial tuberosity

Spiral line

Iliac crest
Hip bone

Anterior gluteal line

Inferior gluteal line
Ischium
Greater trochanter
Neck of femur
Intertrochanteric crest

Lesser trochanter
Gluteal tuberosity

Femur

Linea aspera

Figure 12 Bones of the right hip

The femur has a long and cylindrical diaphysis. Proximally, it has a short neck inclined to the long axis of the bone and an approximately spherical head that sits in the acetabulum of the pelvis. Distally, the femur thickens into the femoral condyles that make up the proximal part of the knee joint. Differences in the bony anatomy of the femur can affect lower extremity movements and, like other lower limb structural abnormalities, are thought to be related to the incidence of overuse injuries of the lower extremity.

The major structural abnormalities of the femur are femoral anteversion and large Q angle. The Q angle expresses the geometric relationship between the pelvis, femur, patella, and tibia in the frontal plane. It is measured as the acute angle between a line drawn from the anterior superior iliac spine of the pelvis to the centre of the patella and a line drawn from the centre of the patella to the tibial tuberosity. It provides an indication of the medial angulation of the femur between the hip joint and the knee joint, which accommodates the difference between the width of the pelvis and the base of support at the feet. This angle is typically higher in women as a result of their wider pelvis relative to femur length. The Q angle is one of the structural measures that have been investigated by sports biomechanists in an attempt to determine the cause of lower extremity overuse injuries, such as those that occur during running.

Femoral anteversion is medial torsion of the femur, the internal rotation of the distal end of the femur relative to the proximal end (see **planes and axes of movement**). This changes the alignment of the bones at the knee and may lead to knee overuse injuries caused by malalignment of the femur relative to the patella and tibia, such as patellofemoral pain. Observing the static standing posture of an individual can identify femoral anteversion; the patella, or kneecap, is turned inwards instead of pointing straight ahead, and the toes are often turned in too. It is possible to correct the anteversion of the femur surgically, although this is only considered if the anteversion is severe enough to interfere with daily activities.

See also: bone; bone classification; hip; hip – joint; hip – ligaments; hip – muscles; lumbar spine and pelvis – muscles.

Hip – Joint

The hip joint is formed between the femur and the hip bone of the pelvis. The hip bone consists of the ilium, ischium, and pubis, which are fused. Both hip bones, along with the sacrum and coccyx of the spine, form the pelvis. Therefore, the hip joint is the link between the pelvis in the torso and the thigh in the lower extremity. The femur is held firmly in place by strong ligaments and the joint capsule. The hip is a ball and socket joint (see **joints**), with the head of the femur fitting into the acetabulum of the hip bone, and is the most mobile joint of the lower extremity. Movements at the hip are sagittal plane flexion-extension, frontal plane abduction-adduction, and transverse plane internal-external rotation (see **planes and axes of movement**).

Because of its high mobility, malalignment of the hip joint can occur during running. This may lead to overuse injuries of the lower extremity because poor alignment at the hip will result in adaptations further down the kinetic chain between the hip and the ground. Incorrect alignment of the lower extremity changes the distribution of load in the bony and soft tissue structures; this is particularly significant as loads of up to three times body weight are transmitted up the lower extremity with each foot strike during running. When we consider that there are around 500 foot strikes with each limb during every mile run, it is easy to appreciate how these small changes can become significant. Common alignment problems at the hip include excessive adduction and excessive internal rotation. Excessive hip adduction is usually due to the pelvis dropping on the contralateral (opposite) side during the stance phase of gait. This may be due to weakness in the ipsilateral hip abductor muscles, but may also be due to a lack of stability in the lower torso, commonly known as core stability (see **Hot Topic 4**).

See also: **hip; hip – bones; hip – ligaments; hip – muscles; joint classification; lumbar spine and pelvis – muscles.**

Hot Topic 4 Core Stability

The core region of the body is the lumbopelvic-hip complex. This includes the lumbar vertebrae, pelvis, hip joints, and the muscles and ligaments that produce or restrict movement of these segments. This area has become the focus of attention in injury prevention and rehabilitation strategies. The main concept of core stability is that the trunk must be stable if the extremities that are attached to it are to be used safely and effectively. It relies mostly on muscular activity to increase trunk and hip stiffness.

The multiple muscles involved in stabilizing the core are in several layers around the abdomen. The muscle fibres in each layer have a different orientation than the other layers. This arrangement provides greater stability at the core than if all the fibres were in the same direction in each layer. As an illustration, the same concept gives a thin sheet of multi-layered plywood its great strength. Core stability develops from the co-contraction of agonist-antagonist muscle groups in each of the three planes of movement. In athletes with a weak core, these core muscles may not be automatically activated to provide trunk stabilization when needed.

While learning to activate the correct muscles, the athlete should sit or lie with the pelvis in a neutral position and think about drawing the navel up and in towards the spine. This is a subtle movement and, therefore, may require a different sort of body awareness than the power athlete is used to. Although the movement is small, it has a significant effect on the stability of the whole body. Another way to determine whether the transverse abdominis is being activated is to locate the place on the front of the pelvis where the muscle can be felt at the surface. On the front of the pelvis are two bony protuberances, the anterior superior iliac spines that can be felt anteriorly just below the top of the iliac crests laterally on the pelvis. Just medial to these bony protuberances is the soft tissue region where the transverse abdominis can be felt. To learn how this muscle feels when activated, an athlete should cough with their fingertips against this region – he or she should feel the muscle tighten and relax. When the transverse abdominis is consciously contracted, the same tension should be felt under the fingertips. This is a good test to use during core stability training to determine whether the correct muscles are being activated.

Further Reading

De Blaiser, C., Roosen, P., Willems, T., Danneels, L., Vanden Bossche, L., & De Ridder, R. (2017). Is core stability a risk factor for lower extremity injuries in an athletic population? A systematic review. *Physical Therapy in Sport, 30,* 48–56.

Hip – Ligaments

The hip is a very stable joint, with stability provided by the ball and socket configuration of the femur and pelvic bones and several thick and strong ligaments (Figure 13). There are three ligaments external to the hip joint: the iliofemoral, ischiofemoral, and pubofemoral ligaments. They are named according to the parts of the hip bone that they are attached to, plus their attachment to the femur. There are two more ligaments at the hip inside the ball and socket of the joint: the ligamentum teres (ligament of the head of the femur) and the transverse acetabular ligament. The ligamentum teres directly attaches the head of the femur to the acetabulum of the hip bone. There is a small pit in the smooth head of the femur, the fovea, where the ligament attaches. Similarly, the other end of the ligament attaches to the centre of the acetabular fossa, where it is surrounded by the smooth lunate surface of the acetabulum. This internal hip joint ligament prevents the head of the femur from rotating too far in any direction within the acetabulum. The transverse acetabular ligament helps to make the socket of the hip joint deeper, along with the acetabular labrum, a rim of fibrocartilage around the edge of the acetabulum. The ligament crosses the acetabular notch, part of the rim not extended by the labrum, making a complete ring of soft tissue. As a result of this extension of the acetabulum, more than half of the femoral head fits within the socket of the hip joint.

As a synovial joint (see **joint classification**), the hip joint is surrounded by a fibrous capsule. Thickenings of this capsule form the three external ligaments of the hip. These ligaments spiral from the pelvis to the femur, providing strong support for the joint. The most anterior ligament is the iliofemoral ligament, also known as the Y-ligament because it has a characteristic inverted Y-shape. This ligament arises from the anterior inferior iliac spine and acetabular rim of the pelvis, winding anteriorly and distally to attach at two points on the intertrochanteric line on the proximal anterior femur. The major role of this ligament is to prevent hyperextension of the hip joint. The pubofemoral ligament has an anteroinferior position. It attaches to the obturator crest, laterally on the pubic bone and runs laterally and distally to blend with the iliofemoral ligament at its femoral attachment. This ligament prevents excessive abduction of the hip joint. The third capsular ligament lies posterior to the hip joint. The ischiofemoral ligament arises from the ischial part of the rim of the acetabulum, spiralling proximally and

(a) Anterior view of cross-section through joint

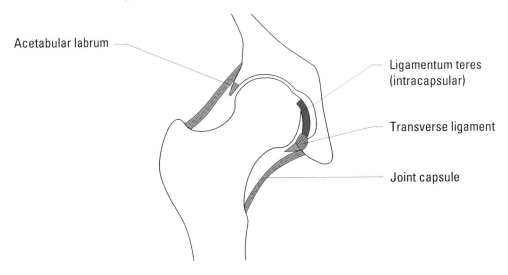

Acetabular labrum

Ligamentum teres
(intracapsular)

Transverse ligament

Joint capsule

(b) Anterior view of intact joint

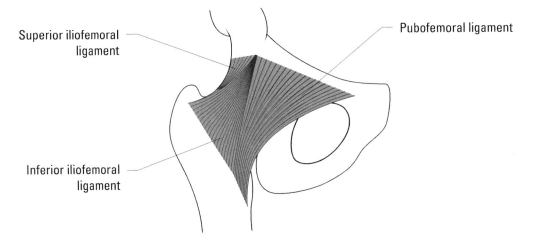

Superior iliofemoral
ligament

Pubofemoral ligament

Inferior iliofemoral
ligament

Figure 13 Ligaments of the right hip. Adapted from Watkins (2014).

laterally to attach to the superior surface of the neck of the femur, just medial to the greater trochanter. This ligament is the weakest of the three. All of the ligaments become tighter during hip extension, preventing hyperextension and pushing the head of the femur into the acetabulum and maximizing the stability of the joint.

Due to the high degree of stability at the hip joint, provided by these strong ligaments which surround the joint as well as the bony structure of the femur and hip bone, the hip joint is rarely dislocated. This is in contrast to the equivalent upper extremity joint, the glenohumeral joint at the shoulder (see **shoulder complex – joints**), which is the most commonly dislocated joint in the body. Both are ball and socket joints, but the glenohumeral joint has a much shallower socket. Since the hip must support and transfer the weight of the entire upper body to the lower extremities during standing and locomotion, this stability is an important feature.

See also: **hip; hip – bones; hip – joint; hip – muscles; lumbar spine and pelvis – muscles.**

Hip – Muscles

The muscles of the thigh can be divided broadly into the anterior femoral muscles on the front of the thigh, and the medial femoral and posterior femoral muscles on the medial side and back of the thigh respectively (Figure 14; Table 4). These muscles have actions at both the knee (see **knee – muscles**) and the hip. This section will focus on the role of the muscles of the thigh in hip rotations.

The muscles on the front of the thigh are the quadriceps femoris group and the sartorius. The quadriceps femoris group consists of rectus femoris and the three vasti: vastus lateralis, vastus medialis, and vastus intermedius. As a whole, the group crosses the front of the knee and extends it; rectus femoris also flexes the hip. The major actions of sartorius are flexing and externally rotating the hip. It also contributes to flexing and internally rotating the knee.

As a group, the medial thigh muscles, gracilis, pectineus, and adductors longus, brevis, and magnus act to adduct the hip (see **planes and axes of movement**). Gracilis also has a role in flexing and internally rotating the knee.

The posterior femoral muscles, also known as the hamstrings, cross the back of both the knee and the hip. Biceps femoris extends the hip and flexes and externally rotates the knee. Semitendinosus also extends the hip and flexes the knee.

(a) Anterior view

(b) Posterior view

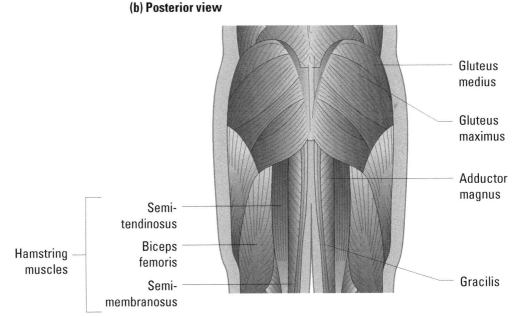

Figure 14 Muscles of the right hip. Adapted from Sewell et al. (2013).

Table 4 Hip muscles contributing to joint movements

Joint movement	Muscles
Hip flexion	Iliopsoas, rectus femoris, sartorius, pectineus, tensor fascia lata
Hip extension	Gluteus maximus, biceps femoris, semitendinosus, semimembranosus
Hip adduction	Adductor longus, adductor magnus, adductor brevis, gracilis, pectineus
Hip abduction	Gluteus medius, gluteus minimus, sartorius
Hip internal rotation	Gluteus medius (anterior portion), gluteus minimus, pectineus
Hip external rotation	Gluteus maximus, sartorius, obturator internus, obturator externus, piriformis, gemellus superior, gemellus inferior, quadratus femoris

The hamstrings consist of biceps femoris, semitendinosus, and semimembranosus. The lateral rotators consist of obturator internus, obturator externus, piriformis, gemellus superior, gemellus inferior, and quadratus femoris.

Additionally, it contributes to internal rotation at the knee. Semimembranosus extends the hip and flexes and internally rotates the knee.

The muscles of the pelvis also contribute to moving the hip joint. The hip extensors on the posterior side of the pelvis are the muscles of the buttocks – gluteus maximus, medius, and minimus – which make up the bulk of this region, plus tensor fasciae latae and the six deep lateral rotators of the thigh – piriformis, the internal and external obturators, gemellus superior and inferior, and quadratus femoris. The action of gluteus maximus is to extend and externally rotate the hip. Through its insertion into the iliotibial band of the thigh, gluteus maximus also stabilizes the knee in extension. The posterior part of the gluteus medius also contributes to these hip movements, but its anterior part flexes the hip and internally rotates it. Gluteus medius also abducts the thigh. The smaller gluteus minimus contributes to flexing, internally rotating, and abducting the thigh.

Given their major contribution to controlling rotations at both the hip and the knee joint, the muscles of the thigh have an important stabilization role during dynamic movements involving the lower extremity. As such, it is important that they are sufficiently strong to fulfil this role and protect and stabilize the joints against the large forces to which they are subjected in sports activities. Examples of compound exercises that engage the muscles of the thigh in their roles at both the hip and the knee are squats, dead lifts, and leg presses.

See also: **hip; hip – bones; hip – joint; hip – ligaments; knee, knee – joint.**

Knee

The knee joint consists of the tibiofemoral joint, which is formed between the distal end of the femur and the proximal end of the tibia, and the patellofemoral joint, between the distal end of the femur and the patella, or kneecap. The major movement at the knee is sagittal plane flexion-extension (see **planes and axes of movement**), with lesser movements in the two secondary planes: abduction-adduction in the frontal plane and internal-external rotation in the transverse plane.

The knee is at risk of both traumatic and overuse injury owing to its structure. The bony surfaces do not provide much stability at the joint. Therefore, the knee relies on soft tissue structures – the cruciate ligaments, collateral ligaments, and menisci – to maintain the joint's integrity. Ligamentous injuries, such as anterior cruciate ligament rupture, are common and often result in residual instability at the knee, even after recovery and rehabilitation (see **In Sports 4**). In individuals who fail to recover fully from a soft tissue injury to the knee, a lack of proprioception often leads to feelings of insecurity about landing, hopping or jumping with the injured leg. The knee may also suffer from unpredictable episodes of 'giving way', which add to feelings of insecurity about relying on that knee. However, this loose-packed arrangement of the joint enables some movement to occur about all three cardinal axes of rotation (see **planes and axes of movement**).

See also: knee – bones; knee – joints; knee – ligaments; knee – muscles.

In Sports 4 Anterior Cruciate Ligament Injury

The anterior cruciate ligament (ACL) is the most commonly injured knee ligament in athletes. The knee is vulnerable to ligament injury because the bone structure does not provide much stability. The rounded condyles of the femur sit on the relatively flat tibial plateau. Additional support is provided at the joint by the menisci and the cruciate and collateral ligaments. The ACL is the primary restraint against anterior tibial displacement and internal rotation of the tibia at the knee. Non-contact ACL injuries occur when a high force at the joint in the direction of either internal rotation or anterior tibial translation exceeds the tensile strength of the ligament. Typically this occurs during landing from a jump or cutting in sports such as basketball, soccer and volleyball. Female athletes are at a much higher risk of ACL injury than their male counterparts. Female athletes may be at up to six times greater risk of ACL injury compared to men playing the same sport at the same level, although more conservative estimates suggest women have about double the risk. The knee is at risk of injury in situations where the foot is fixed on the floor and bearing weight, while the body continues to move. For example, a typical mechanism of ACL injury is landing off balance from a jump and externally rotating the thigh and trunk while the knee is flexed, internally rotated and loaded.

Rupture of the ACL causes knee instability in rotation and anterior translation and abduction laxity. About half of all ACL tears are surgically repaired. Conservative (non-surgical) treatment options are available for those athletes who don't want to return to high level sports, or those who are 'copers' and show no symptoms of instability after rupture of the ligament. In this case, the injury is treated with rehabilitation exercises and the use of knee bracing. Most athletes and other active individuals choose surgical reconstruction of the ACL. The damaged ACL is typically replaced by a section of patellar or hamstrings tendon. This provides a stronger restraint than simply repairing the ruptured ligament. Following surgery, the athlete will spend 6–8 weeks in a knee brace and up to 12 months of rehabilitation before returning to play.

An ACL tear is a devastating season-ending injury for an athlete. For this reason, there has been ongoing interest in the research field to develop and test ACL injury prevention programmes. Injury prevention programmes typically contain one or more of the following components: strengthening, balance, plyometrics, neuromuscular control, technique modification. While several programmes have shown success in research studies, they have yet to be widely incorporated into sports programmes.

Further Reading

Hewett, T. E., Myer, G. D., Ford, K. R., Paterno, M. V., & Quatman, C. E. (2016). Mechanisms, prediction, and prevention of ACL injuries: Cut risk with three sharpened and validated tools. *Journal of Orthopaedic Research, 34*(11), 1843–1855. http://doi.org/10.1002/jor.23414

Knee – Bones

The knee joint has a large sagittal plane range of motion (flexion-extension; see **planes and axes of movement**). The joint is formed between the two major long bones of the lower limb: the tibia, lying between the knee and the ankle, and the femur, lying between the knee and the hip. Although the fibula contributes to the ankle joint, it is not part of the knee joint. However, there is a third bone present at the knee, the patella (kneecap), which forms the patellofemoral joint by running along the intertrochanteric groove in the femur (Figure 15). Stabilization of the joint is predominantly by soft tissue structures – the anterior and posterior cruciate ligaments, the medial and lateral collateral ligaments, and the medial and lateral menisci. The distal end of the femur – the femoral condyles – rests on the flattened tibial plateau.

The primary knee joint axis runs in a mediolateral direction, although its absolute position varies with knee flexion. There are also lesser amounts of rotation in the two secondary planes, with abduction and adduction occurring around the anteroposterior axis and internal and external rotation occurring around the longitudinal axis of the tibia. Historically, these secondary planes of motion have been considered insignificant in the investigation of the cause of overuse injury at the knee. However, as sports biomechanists have access to more advanced equipment for three-dimensional motion analysis (see **Hot Topic 5**), more research has focused on these smaller joint movements. It is hypothesized that slight malalignments in the bones of the lower limb may change the amount and pattern of motion around the secondary axes of rotation at the knee and that these small changes, when repeated over the thousands of repetitions that occur during walking, running or other activities, may contribute to the development of overuse injuries at the joint.

Malalignment of the bones at the knee can lead to osteoarthritic deterioration of the condyles of the joint, with varus (adduction) alignment leading to deterioration of the medial compartment, and valgus (abduction) alignment leading to deterioration of the lateral compartment. Biomechanics researchers are interested in conservative measures to improve the functional ability of individuals with knee osteoarthritis, such as knee braces or in-shoe orthotics to improve the alignment of the bones at the knee joint and reduce the pressure on the arthritic side. These measures can improve quality of life and the ability of a person with osteoarthritis

(a) Anterior view

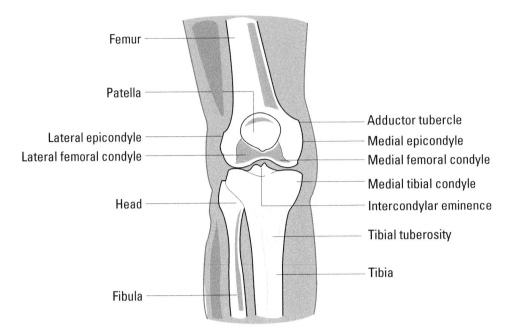

Femur

Patella

Lateral epicondyle

Lateral femoral condyle

Head

Fibula

Adductor tubercle

Medial epicondyle

Medial femoral condyle

Medial tibial condyle

Intercondylar eminence

Tibial tuberosity

Tibia

(b) Posterior view

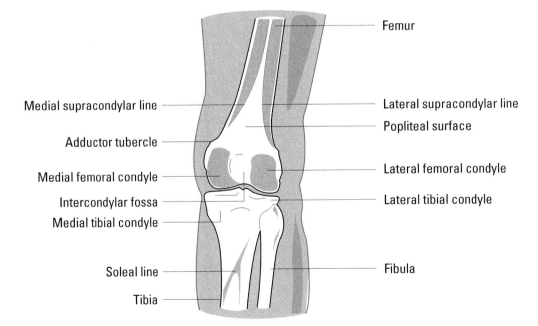

Femur

Medial supracondylar line

Adductor tubercle

Medial femoral condyle

Intercondylar fossa

Medial tibial condyle

Soleal line

Tibia

Lateral supracondylar line

Popliteal surface

Lateral femoral condyle

Lateral tibial condyle

Fibula

Figure 15 Bones of the right knee

to remain physically active, delaying or possibly removing the need for surgery. If knee osteoarthritis progresses beyond the limit at which these conservative measures can provide relief, total knee joint replacement is the surgical option. This involves replacing the distal end of the femur and the proximal end of the tibia with metal and polyethylene components. The prosthesis typically lasts for about 15 years and individuals can return to most sports activities, even skiing, after recovery from surgery.

See also: **bone; bone classification; knee; knee – joints; knee – ligaments; knee – muscles.**

Hot Topic 5 Movement Analysis

Correct technique is a foundation of all athletic activities. Good technique is critical for high performance and to minimize the risk of injury. Traditionally, movement analysis has been mostly qualitative, that is, directly observing athletic activities as they happen and describing them, but not making direct measurements. With practice, a trained eye can determine gross changes in an athlete's technique and locate the joint or segment of the body that is affected. This method is quick and requires no special equipment but relies heavily on the skill of the observer. These days, however, everyone has a video camera available via smartphones and tablets. As a result, the use of video analysis of movement has exploded.

Video analysis is easy to do and has many advantages over direct observation by eye. Perhaps most importantly, a permanent record of the movement of interest is obtained, which can be returned to and reassessed at a future date. The ability to pause and play back the recorded movement at slow speeds is another huge advantage over observational analysis, as it often reveals movements that are either too subtle or occur too quickly to be registered by the naked eye. However, video analysis also has its limitations, the most significant of which is its two-dimensionality. In recording movement onto video, a three-dimensional activity is projected onto a two-dimensional plane. Consequently, movements toward and away from or in and out of the plane of view of the camera are difficult to detect and assess. The impact of the two-dimensionality of video analysis is greatest in sports skills with a large amount of rotation between body segments, such as pitching or a golf swing. Many apps are available to assist with video analysis of athletic movements, some even offer the ability to measure angles. However, a major caution must be given here: the angles measured are of a two-dimensional projection onto the video screen of a three-dimensional movement. If any parts of the body are not fully in the plane of the camera throughout the movement, the angle measured will not be the true angle the joint was positioned in. This can be highly misleading and lead to incorrect conclusions about the performance.

The most sophisticated type of movement analysis is three-dimensional kinematic and kinetic analysis. Such an assessment requires advanced motion capture and force-measuring equipment and a skilled biomechanist to collect high quality data and interpret it appropriately using evidence from the research literature and biomechanical principles. Three-dimensional motion analysis is also more time-consuming, both in preparing athletes for their movement skill to be recorded and during the data analysis and interpretation. Consequently, it is also more expensive than video analysis. However, a three-dimensional movement analysis provides comprehensive and objective quantitative information about the movement performance. All of this information can be interpreted by the skilled sports biomechanist and used as the basis for an assessment focused on improving performance and/or reducing injury risk.

Further Reading

Knudson, D. V. (2013). *Qualitative diagnosis of human movement: Improving performance in sport and exercise* (3rd ed.). Champaign, IL: Human Kinetics.

Milner, C. E. (2018). Motion analysis using online systems. In C. Payton & R. Bartlett (Eds.), *Biomechanical analysis of movement in sport and exercise: The British Association of Sport and Exercise Sciences guide* (2nd ed.). London: Routledge.

Knee – Joints

The knee consists of the tibiofemoral joint between the long bones of the lower extremity, where the femoral condyles articulate with the tibial plateau. The patellofemoral joint lies between the intertrochanteric groove of the femur and the patella (kneecap). The primary movement at the knee is flexion-extension in the sagittal plane (see **planes and axes of movement**). Typically, the knee has a range of motion of about 140° of flexion-extension, from about 5° of hyperextension to 135° of flexion. Secondary movements at the knee are abduction-adduction and internal-external rotation.

The secondary planes of motion at the knee joint are of interest to researchers who are trying to determine the biomechanical causes of overuse injuries to the knee, such as patellofemoral pain and iliotibial band syndrome. Although the movements in the secondary planes are smaller than the flexion-extension motion, when minor deviations in these movements are repeated over and over, as in walking or running, the effects may accumulate and contribute to overuse injury. Other factors thought to be related to overuse injuries at the knee are malalignment at the hip joint or in the foot.

The knee joint is susceptible to traumatic ligament tears because it relies on soft tissue and not bony structures for its stability. The most common acute injury at the knee joint is a tear of the anterior cruciate ligament (ACL: see **In Sports 2**).

It should be noted that the terms flexion and extension at the knee refer to rotation in the opposite direction about the mediolateral axis of the joint than at other joints. Flexion is generally the sagittal plane rotation that brings the distal segment towards the proximal segment anteriorly about the mediolateral axis in the **anatomical position**. However, flexion of the knee, brought about mainly by the hamstrings on the back of the thigh, is movement of the leg towards the hamstrings posteriorly. Contrast this with flexion of the hip by rectus femoris on the front of the thigh: movement of the thigh towards the front of the thorax.

See also: **bone; bone classification; knee; knee – bones; knee – joints; knee – ligaments; knee – muscles.**

Knee – Ligaments

The knee relies heavily on its ligaments for stability, since the bones themselves are somewhat flat in the area of contact. There are four major ligaments at the tibiofemoral joint, plus the menisci – additional soft tissue structures that also provide stability at the knee (Figure 16). The patellofemoral joint has one ligament associated with it: the patellar ligament.

The four ligaments associated with the tibiofemoral joint are in two pairs. Inside the joint are the anterior and posterior cruciate ligaments (ACL, PCL), and outside the joint are the medial and lateral collateral ligaments (MCL, LCL). Each ligament checks extremes of different rotations at the knee, according to its orientation and attachments. The ACL is the most commonly injured knee ligament in athletes, and is typically injured in a non-contact situation (see **In Sports 4**). The two cruciate ligaments are so named because they run on opposite diagonals in the middle of the knee joint, crossing over each other and making an X shape. The ACL runs in a posterolateral direction from the anterior portion of the intercondylar area of the tibia to the medial side of the lateral femoral condyle. The PCL runs anteromedially from the posterior part of the tibial intercondylar area to the lateral side of the medial condyle of the femur. The primary roles of the ACL and PCL are to prevent anterior and posterior sliding of the tibia respectively. Since the tibial plateau is relatively flat, this is important in maintaining the integrity of the joint when muscle action tends to translate the tibia on the femur. The cruciate ligaments also check axial rotation of the tibia, with the ACL checking internal rotation and the PCL external rotation.

The MCL and LCL ligaments lie outside the joint capsule on the medial and lateral aspects of the knee. The MCL runs from the medial epicondyle of the femur to the medial condyle of the tibia and the LCL runs from the lateral epicondyle of the femur to the head of the fibula. Together these two ligaments check hyperextension of the knee. Individually, the MCL and LCL prevent excessive abduction and adduction of the knee respectively. Injury to the collateral ligaments typically occurs in sports activities as a result of contact. For example, the LCL could be injured during a heavy tackle from the side in rugby when the legs of the player being tackled are obstructed and prevented from moving with the tackle by a teammate lying on the ground. As the tackler moves the upper body of the player sideways, the collateral ligaments that oppose the movement are under

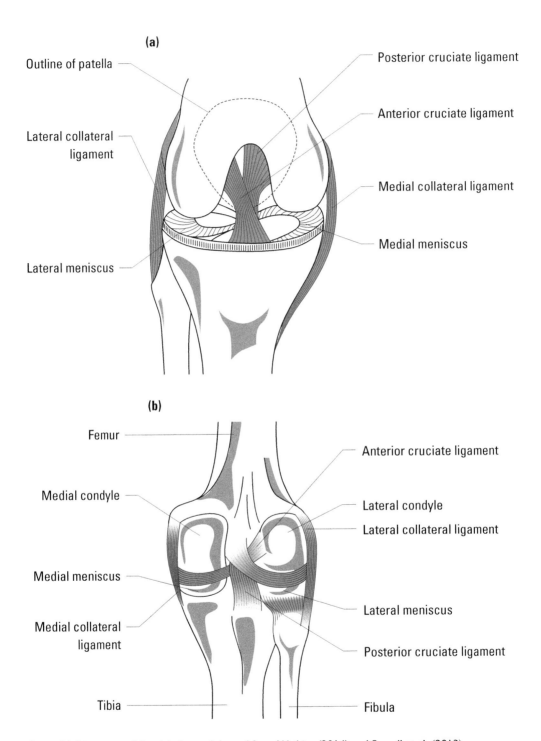

Figure 16 Ligaments of the right knee. Adapted from Watkins (2014) and Sewell et al. (2013).

tensile strain. If the large force being applied during the tackle is greater than the tensile strength of the LCL when the knee is being forcibly adducted, the ligament will rupture. At the moment the ligament ruptures, a loud pop is often heard as the ligament snaps. The result is an immediate loss of stability at the knee, allowing it to move into an extreme adducted position. The damaged ligament is typically surgically repaired or reconstructed in athletes to enable them to regain stability and return to play after a lengthy rehabilitation period.

In addition to these ligaments, the medial and lateral tibial condyles each have a meniscus. This is a C-shaped ring of fibrocartilage around the edge of each condyle which helps to deepen the tibial plateau and provide additional support and stability at the joint. The menisci increase the contact area between the femur and tibia, helping to distribute the loads transmitted through the knee more evenly.

Finally, the patellofemoral joint also has a ligament. This joint is different than the tibiofemoral joint because the patella is a sesamoid bone: a bone that lies within a tendon. The patella lies within the tendon of the powerful quadriceps muscle. This tendon crosses the knee joint to attach to the tibia; the patella improves the mechanical advantage of the quadriceps by moving the tendon further away from the centre of the knee joint. The portion of tendon between the quadriceps muscle and the patella is called the quadriceps tendon and the portion below the patella that inserts onto the tibial tuberosity is the patellar tendon.

See also: knee; knee – bones; knee – joints; knee – muscles.

Knee – Muscles

The muscles of the knee are responsible for flexing and extending the joint and for dynamic stabilization of the joint during activity (Figure 17; Table 5). Therefore, these muscles work eccentrically and isometrically as well as concentrically (see **skeletal muscle contraction – types**). The muscle group on the front of the thigh, the quadriceps femoris, is responsible for extending the knee; the muscle group on the back of the thigh, the hamstrings, is responsible for flexing the knee. Other muscles of the lower limb play minor roles in the control of the knee joint. The role of the knee joint during gait provides a good example of the multifunctional roles of the muscles of the knee, with the muscles undergoing concentric and eccentric contraction during various phases of the gait cycle.

(a) Anterior view

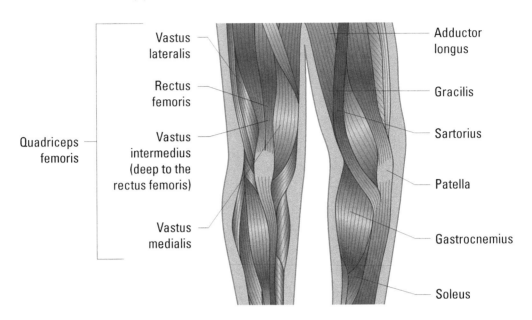

Vastus lateralis

Rectus femoris

Quadriceps femoris

Vastus intermedius (deep to the rectus femoris)

Vastus medialis

Adductor longus

Gracilis

Sartorius

Patella

Gastrocnemius

Soleus

(b) Posterior view

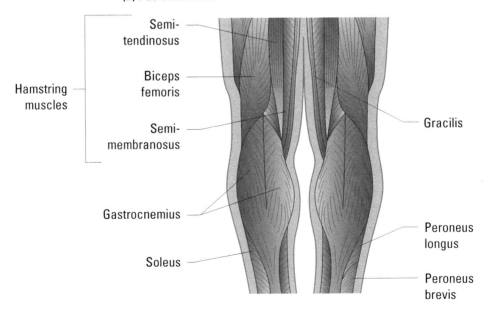

Semi-tendinosus

Biceps femoris

Hamstring muscles

Semi-membranosus

Gastrocnemius

Soleus

Gracilis

Peroneus longus

Peroneus brevis

Figure 17 Muscles of the right knee. Adapted from Sewell et al. (2013).

Table 5 Knee muscles contributing to joint movements

Joint movement	Muscles
Knee flexion	Biceps femoris, semitendinosus, semimembranosus, gastrocnemius, sartorius, gracilis, popliteus
Knee extension	Quadriceps femoris
Knee internal rotation	Semimembranosus, semitendinosus, gracilis, popliteus
Knee external rotation	Biceps femoris

The hamstrings consist of biceps femoris, semitendinosus, and semimembranosus. The quadriceps femoris consist of rectus femoris, vastus lateralis, vastus intermedius, and vastus medialis.

The quadriceps femoris muscle group – the rectus femoris, vastus lateralis, vastus medialis, and vastus intermedius – extends the knee. The hamstrings – the long and short head of the biceps femoris, plus semitendinosus and semimembranosus – flex the knee. Popliteus is a small muscle that flexes and internally rotates the knee. The gastrocnemius of the leg also has a flexing action on the knee, but its major role at the knee is preventing hyperextension of the knee joint. Gastrocnemius also plantarflexes the ankle (see **ankle and foot – muscles**).

During gait, these muscle groups act both concentrically and eccentrically. During the stance phase of walking the knee is flexed. However, there is a tendency for the knee to continue to flex and, ultimately, collapse under the weight of the body. To prevent this, the quadriceps muscle group acts eccentrically to restrict the knee flexion that occurs and ensure that the stance leg is stable while the whole of the body's weight is on it during single limb stance. Similarly, at the end of the swing phase of gait, when the knee is extending to place the foot in front of the body at heel strike, the hamstrings are acting eccentrically to slow the speed at which the knee is extending and prevent hyperextension of the joint from occurring. The hamstrings act concentrically at the end of the stance phase and beginning of the swing phase of gait to flex the knee in preparation for the swing limb moving forward past the stance limb.

The muscles of the knee provide support for the joint during dynamic activity (**Hot Topic 6**). Since the knee joint is stabilized by soft tissue structures rather than its bony architecture, it is vital that these muscles have sufficient strength to support the joint during sporting activities. To isolate these specific muscle groups, single joint exercises should be used. For example, the seated knee extension exercise isolates the quadriceps muscle group, whereas the standing or lying hamstring curl isolates the hamstrings. However, the muscle groups rarely work in isolation in a sports movement, so compound or multi-joint exercises reflect the functional role of the muscles more appropriately. Examples of compound exercises that work the muscles of the knee include squats of all types, dead lifts, leg presses, and power cleans.

Further Reading

Levine, D., Richards, J., & Whittle, M. W. (Eds.) (2012). *Whittle's gait analysis* (5th ed.), Oxford: Churchill Livingstone Elsevier.

See also: **knee; knee – bones; knee – joints; knee – ligaments.**

Hot Topic 6 Wearable Activity Trackers

There has been an explosion of options for wearable activity trackers in the past few years. Wearable devices have gone from something that might be worn by athletes during training to monitor a single metric, such as heart rate monitors, to devices that track and record multiple metrics, including heart rate, number of steps, calories burned, stair climbing, and sleep time, 24 hours a day, 7 days a week. The cost of these devices is now within reach of most people and by downloading the tracked data directly to smartphone apps, we have instant access to more data about our activity than ever before. The great opportunity with wearable activity trackers is that they get the general public interested in their daily activity levels and provide an easy way to set personal goals to improve health. Most apps also contain a social component that enables users to set and join group challenges – either with friends or as part of a growing online community. In a world where obesity is rampant and children are developing lifestyle diseases previously only seen in adults approaching middle age, the potential of these wearable devices to stimulate an interest in physical activity is extremely important.

However, there are some potential pitfalls in the output data provided by activity trackers. Heart rate monitoring technology has been around for years and is typically quite accurate. For step count, patterns recorded by accelerometers within a device are processed to estimate when a step occurred. When walking at moderate to fast speeds, steps can be identified quite well. However, step counters tend to struggle at slow walking speeds to differentiate the steps from other non-stepping movements, and steps may be missed. Some metrics are estimated – notably calories burned. Activity trackers take several inputs, likely including the user's height, weight, age, heart rate during activity, and use proprietary algorithms to estimate the energy expenditure and report calories burned. This may provide an estimate that is fairly accurate for some people, but may be off the mark and either too high or too low for others. There is such a wide range of variation among people in terms of body composition, history of physical activity, current fitness level, efficiency of movement, and so on that it is hard to make one-size-fits-all estimates. This is also true for exercise machines, such as treadmills, elliptical trainers, and exercise bikes that estimate calories burned. These limitations may not be of great concern to casual users, but could be critical where high precision is needed, such as for research studies.

The technology of activity tracking is constantly under development and manufacturers compete to provide new features for the consumer. When sedentary behaviour, overweight, and obesity are at epidemic proportions, using technology to make participating in physical activity fun for people who aren't habitually active is a great positive step. But, as with all sources of data, it is important to understand the potential for error in various metrics.

Further Reading

Evenson, K. R., Goto, M. M., & Furberg, R. D. (2015). Systematic review of the validity and reliability of consumer-wearable activity trackers. *International Journal of Behavioral Nutrition and Physical Activity*, 12, 159.

Lumbar Spine and Pelvis

The pelvis is the link between the torso and the lower extremities and the lumbar spine is responsible for movement in this region. The pelvis is a rigid ring made up of several bones, some of which are fused and none of which allow more than a negligible amount of motion between their articulations. The five lumbar vertebrae allow a large range of extension in the lower back and a lesser range of flexion. As with all spinal motion, the movements between adjacent vertebrae are small, but the total for the five vertebrae becomes appreciable.

Since it is the link between the upper and lower body, this region is subject to large forces as movements are transferred between the upper and lower limbs. For example, in rowing, forces generated at the feet against the foot plate must be transferred through the trunk to the hands on the oar to propel the oar through the water. This transfer of energy requires a strong and rigid trunk that will transfer and not absorb the power generated by the lower limbs. The lumbar spine is subjected to high loads during these activities. More importantly in terms of injury risk, it may also be in a weakened position because it can accommodate alignment faults elsewhere in the body to place the lower extremities where they need to be.

Further Reading

Wilson, F., Gissane, C., & McGregor, A. (2014). Ergometer training volume and previous injury predict back pain in rowing: Strategies for injury prevention and rehabilitation. *British Journal of Sports Medicine, 48*, 1534–1537.

See also: lumbar spine and pelvis – bones; lumbar spine and pelvis – joints; lumbar spine and pelvis – ligaments; lumbar spine and pelvis – muscles.

Lumbar Spine and Pelvis – Bones

The pelvis is the junction between the trunk and the lower extremities. It supports the spine and rests on the lower limbs. The pelvis is strong and sturdy and is made up of four bones: the two hip bones, plus the sacrum and coccyx of the distal spine (Figure 18). The bones form a ring with a large aperture in the middle; in women, this aperture is the birth canal. The hip bones themselves are made up of three fused bones: the ilium, ischium, and pubis. The lumbar spine sits immediately

(a) Anterior view

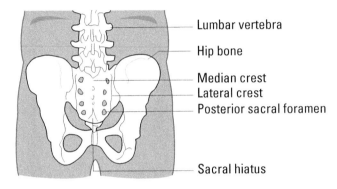

Lumbar vertebra

Sacral promontory
Iliac fossa
Sacrum
Anterior superior iliac spine
Anterior inferior iliac spine
Coccyx
Ischium

Anterior sacral foramen

Saroiliac joint
Hip bone

Acetabulum
Pubis
Pubic
symphysis

(b) Posterior view

Lumbar vertebra

Hip bone

Median crest
Lateral crest
Posterior sacral foramen

Sacral hiatus

(c) Lateral view

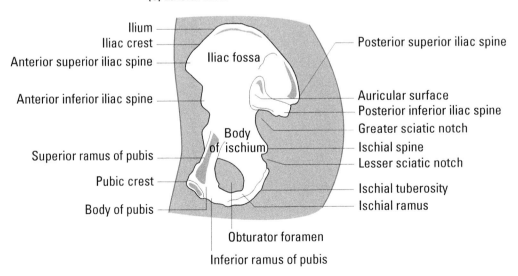

Ilium
Iliac crest
Anterior superior iliac spine

Iliac fossa

Anterior inferior iliac spine

Body
of ischium

Superior ramus of pubis

Pubic crest

Body of pubis

Posterior superior iliac spine

Auricular surface
Posterior inferior iliac spine
Greater sciatic notch
Ischial spine
Lesser sciatic notch

Ischial tuberosity
Ischial ramus

Obturator foramen

Inferior ramus of pubis

Figure 18 Bones of the lumbar spine and pelvis

on top of the sacrum and comprises five individual vertebrae. There are several differences in structure between the male and female pelvis. Most notably, the female pelvis has a wider and more rounded pubic arch.

The pelvis consists of several articulations, between the sacrum and the ilium, the sacrum and the coccyx, and between the pubic bones. However, only very limited movement occurs between the sacrum and the coccyx, at the sacrococcygeal joint, and between the two pubic bones at the pubic symphysis. The lumbar spine is the most mobile part of this region, primarily in extension and flexion.

The pelvic region is a site of overuse injuries. In particular, stress fractures of the pelvis occur in runners. The exact mechanism of these fractures is unclear. Why, for example, do some runners suffer stress fractures more distally in the lower extremity whereas, in other cases, forces are transmitted up through the lower extremity without injury to its tissues and cause a stress fracture in the pelvis? Stress fractures developed through running can occur in most of the bones of the lower extremity and the reasons why they manifest themselves in different places in different runners are the subject of ongoing research in sports biomechanics. Sports biomechanics researchers use advanced techniques, such as three-dimensional motion analysis (see **Hot Topic 5**), to investigate these relationships and have been studying the interrelationships between anatomical, physiological, and training factors and the occurrence of overuse injuries in running for more than 20 years.

Another group of athletes at risk of overuse injury in the lumbar and pelvic region are rowers, who commonly suffer from low back pain. Relationships between the dynamic position of the lumbar spine during rowing and low back pain have also been the subject of investigation by sports biomechanists and physiotherapists in recent years (see **lumbar spine and pelvis – joints**).

See also: hip – joint; **lumbar spine and pelvis; lumbar spine and pelvis – ligaments; lumbar spine and pelvis – muscles; vertebral structure.**

Lumbar Spine and Pelvis – Joints

This region consists of the five lumbar vertebrae and the pelvis. The pelvis is made up of the two hip bones and the sacrum and coccyx of the spine. The pelvis itself is quite rigid and movements between its bones are minimal. However, the lumbar spine has a large extension motion and a more limited amount of flexion, both of which are the sum of relatively small movements at each intervertebral joint.

Acute injuries to the lower back can occur in many sports and are often related to the ballistic (explosive) movements involved. The lower back is particularly vulnerable when it is hyperextended, laterally flexed, and rotated and has a load applied to it. For example, in racquet sports, serving and playing shots while the spine is in this position can lead to muscular strains in the lower back. Weight lifting and weight training also place the back at risk of injury, particularly when heavy lifts are involved. Back injuries are often associated with poor technique or trying to lift too heavy a weight. Among the most common back injuries are spondylolysis (stress fracture of the vertebral arch), spondylosis (degeneration of an intervertebral disc) and spondylolisthesis (anterior misalignment of a vertebra resulting from a bilateral spondylolysis).

Rowers are at risk of overuse injury in this region of the back. Low back pain is common in rowers. Relationships between the dynamic position of the lumbar spine during the rowing movement and low back pain have been the subject of investigation by sports biomechanists and physiotherapists in recent years. However, as with running overuse injuries, it remains unclear which factors are most important in this injury and, therefore, which individuals are most at risk of injury. Possible causes of injury include hip flexor tightness and lack of hip joint flexibility. During the rowing stroke, forward flexion of the trunk should be achieved by hip flexion with the pelvis held in a neutral position with respect to the trunk. However, a lack of flexibility in this region leads to increased posterior pelvic tilt and, consequently, the necessary forward flexion is achieved through the next available structure with sufficient range of motion – the lumbar spine. The following simple hamstring length test can be used to determine whether rowers have sufficient hamstring flexibility to be able to achieve the forward position of the trunk from hip flexion alone. With the athlete lying on their back, with the pelvis neutral, raise the straight leg into as much hip flexion as possible without losing the neutral tilt of the pelvis. If the leg reaches a vertical position – 90° hip flexion – the movement can be achieved. If the rower fails to reach this position, hamstring tightness is restricting their ability to achieve trunk forward lean using the correct and safest technique.

See also: **lumbar spine and pelvis; lumbar spine and pelvis – bones; lumbar spine and pelvis – ligaments; lumbar spine and pelvis – muscles.**

Lumbar Spine and Pelvis – Ligaments

The lumbar spine and pelvis support and transmit the weight of the upper body to the lower extremities. The pelvis has a limited amount of movement between its bones and is supported by strong ligaments. The sacroiliac joint has a very limited amount of movement and is supported by the strong posterior and interosseous sacroiliac ligaments, plus the thinner anterior sacroiliac ligament. The interosseous ligaments are the primary structures involved in the transfer of upper body weight to the pelvis and then to the lower extremities. Movement at the sacroiliac joint is further held in check by the strong sacrotuberous ligaments. These ligaments run from the sacrum to the ischial tuberosity of the pelvis and prevent superior rotation of the inferior end of the sacrum. The lumbosacral joint is supported by the iliolumbar ligaments which run from the transverse processes of the L5 vertebra to the iliac bones of the pelvis. There is also a joint between the sacrum and coccyx, although it does not contribute to weight transfer to the lower extremities. The sacrococcygeal joint is supported by anterior and posterior sacrococcygeal ligaments, which run longitudinally from the sacrum to the coccyx.

The lumbar spine is the distal end of the mobile portion of the vertebral column. The vertebral bodies are large and strong and the articular facets are oriented obliquely to prevent intervertebral rotation movements. The lumbar spine has a large flexion-extension range of motion and is supported by the common longitudinally running ligaments of the vertebral column (see **thoracic region – ligaments**). The strong and wide anterior longitudinal ligament runs the length of the vertebral column and is attached to the anterior surface of the vertebral bodies and intervertebral discs; it helps to prevent hyperextension of the vertebral column. The thinner and weaker posterior longitudinal ligament is attached to the posterior surface of the intervertebral discs and lies inside the vertebral canal. The posterior wall of the vertebral canal is formed by the ligamentum flavum, which connects adjacent vertebral arches at the laminae. The remaining ligaments connect the various processes of the vertebrae. The interspinous ligaments lie between adjacent spinous processes and weakly connect them. The strong supraspinous ligament connects the tips of the spinous processes and helps to prevent hyperflexion. There are also thin and weak intertransverse ligaments in the lumbar region which connect adjacent transverse processes.

See also: lumbar spine and pelvis; lumbar spine and pelvis – bones; lumbar spine and pelvis – joints; lumbar spine and pelvis – muscles.

Lumbar Spine and Pelvis – Muscles

The muscles of the lumbar spine contribute to flexing and extending the lower back, and also play a key role in postural support and stability (Table 6). The muscles of the pelvis can be divided broadly into those that flex the hip and those that extend the hip (see Figure 24) (see **hip – muscles**).

The posterior lumbar spine region contains the quadratus lumborum and erector spinae. which extend the lumbar spine and flex it laterally. Spine extension occurs when the muscles on both sides of the posterior trunk contract; lateral flexion occurs when only the muscles on the side that the trunk is flexed towards contract. The front of the lumbar spine and pelvic region is the distal part of the abdomen and contains the internal and external obliques, transverse abdominals, rectus abdominis, and the small pyramidalis. These anterior muscles hold the abdominal organs in place, flex the trunk anteriorly and laterally, and rotate it about its long axis. The transverse abdominals are major postural muscles and have received a lot of attention as a result of the key role they play in stabilizing the spine during many sports movements; both to protect the spine and to enable power transfer between body segments (see **Hot Topic 4**).

The lumbar spine and pelvis are often involved in overuse injuries in sport. Low back pain is a common complaint in elite athletes and recreational sports people alike. Although the immediate pain usually resolves with rest, like most overuse injuries, the problem will return unless the root cause is determined and rectified.

Table 6 Lumbar spine and pelvis muscles contributing to joint movements

Joint movement	Muscles
Lumbar flexion	Both*: rectus abdominis, internal obliques, external obliques
Lumbar extension	Both*: quadratus lumborum, iliocostalis, longissimus, spinalis
Lateral flexion to the right**	Right: quadratus lumborum, iliocostalis, longissimus, spinalis, external oblique, internal oblique

Notes: * Both indicates this is the action when both muscles contract together.

** A direction is given for lateral flexion and rotation to illustrate whether the individual muscle on the same or opposite side to the direction of movement is active.

The erector spinae consists of iliocostalis, longissimus, and spinalis.

For example, in those sports that require a large anterior pelvic tilt to be maintained for long periods, the muscles responsible for this movement, mainly psoas major on the front of the pelvis, can become chronically shortened and prevent normal pelvic tilt from being achieved in the normal standing posture. Examples of such sports are rowing and cycling. However, low back problems can also occur in runners, since they need to maintain correct trunk and upper body posture while supporting themselves alternately on opposite legs during the running stride. This problem builds up slowly over a long time and the subtle change in posture may not be detected until it becomes severe enough to cause low back problems. For the trunk and upper body to remain upright in a standing position, the lumbar spine must hyperextend into increased lumbar lordosis to counteract the increased anterior tilt of the pelvis. Although this compensation does enable the upper trunk to maintain its normal position with respect to the rest of the body, it overloads the lumbar spine and predisposes it to overuse injury and the onset of low back pain.

A lordotic posture can be recognized by the increased concavity of the lower back when viewed from the side. The pelvic tilt can be estimated by measuring the angle between the horizontal and a line between the posterior superior iliac spines and the anterior superior iliac spines of the pelvis in the sagittal plane (see **planes and axes of movement**). In a normal standing posture with the pelvis held in a neutral position by the surrounding musculature, this measure of anterior pelvic tilt will be approximately 10°. With increased anterior tilt as described above, this value will increase with greater inclination of the pelvis. Once this root cause of the problem is recognized, remedial measures can be put in place to lengthen the hip flexor muscles of the pelvis and retrain the individual to recognize and maintain a neutral alignment of the pelvis and strengthen the associated postural muscles appropriately.

The gluteal muscles on the rear of the pelvis are well developed in sprint athletes such as track sprint runners and track cyclists. In these sports, the hip needs to be actively extended during every cycle of the running stride or pedal stroke. In sprint runners, these muscles are actively contracted to bring the body forwards over the standing leg during the stance phase of the running cycle. This is a closed chain movement of hip extension, with the lower extremity in fixed contact with the ground and the body moving forward over it. In cycling, approximately half of the circular motion of the pedal stroke involves extending the hip from a flexed position.

Strengthening muscles in this region takes several different forms. The large gluteal muscles can be developed effectively by weight training exercises of various types. Single joint exercises that isolate hip extension can be used, but compound exercises that involve all of the joints of the lower extremity might reflect more appropriately how the muscles are required to perform during sports activity. For example, in sports such as cycling and rowing, hip extension and knee extension occur simultaneously. This action is replicated during weight training by various squatting exercises. The postural muscles of the lumbar spine are trained and developed by more subtle means, such as locating and then maintaining the correct pelvic orientation. Supplementary techniques such as yoga and Pilates can be effective for this kind of strengthening.

See also: **core stability; hip; hip – joint; hip – muscles; lumbar spine and pelvis; lumbar spine and pelvis – bones; lumbar spine and pelvis – joints; lumbar spine and pelvis – ligaments.**

Shoulder Complex

The shoulder complex consists of the glenohumeral, acromioclavicular and scapulothoracic joints. The glenohumeral joint is formed between the proximal end of the humerus and the glenoid fossa of the scapula (the shoulder blade). It is a ball and socket joint (see **joints**) but, since the glenoid fossa is shallow, it relies on ligamentous and tendinous attachments to maintain its integrity and prevent dislocation. Owing to the structure of the joint, the shoulder is capable of movement in all three cardinal planes: flexion-extension, abduction-adduction, and internal-external rotation, plus the combined movement of circumduction (see **planes and axes of movement**). The range of motion of the glenohumeral joint is increased by movements at the scapulothoracic joint. Movement of the scapula on the back of the thoracic cage alters the position of the glenoid fossa and enables a greater range of motion to occur at the shoulder. This relationship is known as 'scapulohumeral rhythm'.

Due to its structure, the shoulder is a flexible joint capable of manoeuvring the arm and hand into a huge range of positions. However, this flexibility also puts the joint at risk of injury. Since the stability and integrity of the joint are maintained by soft tissue structures rather than bony anatomy, the soft tissues can be damaged if the load applied to them is too great. The shoulder is at risk of both traumatic and overuse injury. A typical traumatic injury is dislocation of the head of the humerus from the glenoid fossa of the scapula. This injury is relatively common in contact sports such as rugby, when contact with another player or the ground can result in a blow to the shoulder that is severe enough to force the humerus out of its shallow socket. Overuse injuries occur when a lower load is applied to the joint, but is applied repeatedly during the course of training and competition. Although such a load poses no threat to the integrity of the joint during an isolated episode of loading, the cumulative effects can cause sufficient microtrauma to damage the tissue faster than it can be repaired. An example of this type of injury is swimmer's shoulder, or subacromial impingement syndrome (see **shoulder complex – joints**).

See also: **shoulder complex – bones; shoulder complex – joints; shoulder complex – ligaments; shoulder complex – muscles.**

Shoulder Complex – Bones

The shoulder is the most proximal joint of the upper extremity and has the greatest multiaxial range of motion of all the upper extremity joints. The glenohumeral joint is formed between the scapula (the shoulder blade) and the humerus, the long bone in the upper arm that contributes to both the shoulder and the elbow joint (Figure 19). The glenohumeral joint is a ball and socket joint and, as such, makes the arm very mobile with respect to the torso. The joint has only a shallow socket in the glenoid fossa of the scapula for the humerus to sit in, but is protected against displacement by strong ligament and tendinous attachments. The shoulder complex comprises the glenohumeral joint plus the acromioclavicular joint, between the scapula and the lateral end of the clavicle (the collarbone), and the scapulothoracic joint, between the subscapular fossa and the thoracic cage. The scapulothoracic joint is not a traditional joint, since bone does not articulate directly with bone (see **joint classification**). However, this structure makes a large contribution to the mobility of the shoulder complex.

The humerus is the longest bone of the upper limb and consists of a long diaphysis with a hemispherical head proximally at the shoulder joint. Distally the bone thickens out into the articular condyles that form the proximal part of the elbow joint. Overuse injuries of the upper extremity are less common than in the lower extremity, since the upper body is not subjected as frequently to high repetitions with high loading. However, overuse injuries of the upper extremity do occur in throwing and hitting sports and those that involve repetitive stereotyped movements; particularly at the glenohumeral joint, which relies heavily on soft tissue structures to maintain its integrity (see **shoulder complex – joints**). Traumatic injuries to the bones of the shoulder are relatively common and typically result from a fall.

A common traumatic injury to the clavicle is fracture of the lateral or middle third of the bone. The most common mechanism of fracture is falling onto the outstretched arm and hand or directly onto the end of the shoulder. This particular injury may appear to be relatively minor, but it has the potential for serious complications because several important structures lie just below the bone: the top of the lung, the subclavian blood vessels, and a nervous structure known as the brachial plexus. To minimize the risk of this injury, learning how to fall properly in contact sports such as rugby and judo is essential and should be taught from the earliest stage of player development.

(a) Anterior view

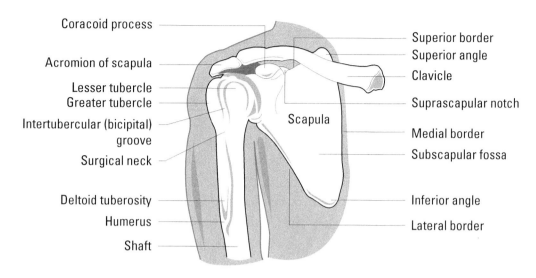

Coracoid process

Acromion of scapula

Lesser tubercle
Greater tubercle

Intertubercular (bicipital) groove

Surgical neck

Deltoid tuberosity

Humerus

Shaft

Scapula

Superior border
Superior angle

Clavicle

Suprascapular notch

Medial border

Subscapular fossa

Inferior angle

Lateral border

(b) Posterior view

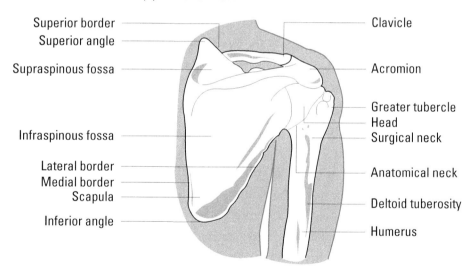

Superior border
Superior angle

Supraspinous fossa

Infraspinous fossa

Lateral border
Medial border
Scapula

Inferior angle

Clavicle

Acromion

Greater tubercle
Head
Surgical neck

Anatomical neck

Deltoid tuberosity

Humerus

Figure 19 Bones of the right shoulder

Another traumatic shoulder injury common to those contact sports is shoulder subluxation, or partial dislocation, more accurately described as acromioclavicular joint sprain. This injury tends to occur when the athlete falls directly onto the end of the shoulder. The severity of the injury depends on how much of the ligamentous structure spanning the joint is disrupted (see **shoulder complex – ligaments**).

See also: **bone; bone classification; shoulder complex; shoulder complex – joint; shoulder complex – ligaments; shoulder complex – muscles.**

Shoulder Complex – Joints

The shoulder complex has three individual joints, involving the scapula (the shoulder blade) clavicle (the collarbone), and the humerus. The glenohumeral joint is the most proximal joint of the upper extremity and has the greatest multiaxial range of motion of all the upper extremity joints. It is formed between the glenoid fossa of the scapula and the proximal end of the humerus. The shoulder joint is a ball and socket joint (see **joints**) and, as such, makes the arm very mobile in relation to the torso. The joint has only a shallow socket formed by the glenoid fossa of the scapula, against which the hemispherical head of the humerus sits; it is protected against dislocation by strong ligament and tendinous attachments. This arrangement enables the large ranges of motion at the joint but also puts it at greater risk of dislocation than the comparable lower extremity joint, the hip joint, which has a much deeper ball and socket and is, consequently, dislocated much less often. Movements possible at the glenohumeral joint are flexion, extension, abduction, adduction, internal rotation, external rotation, horizontal adduction and horizontal abduction (see **planes and axes of movement**). Horizontal abduction and adduction are movements that occur only at the glenohumeral joint. The movements occur in the transverse plane, with horizontal adduction being movement towards the midline in this plane and horizontal abduction being movement away from the midline.

The two other joints of the shoulder complex are the acromioclavicular joint, between the lateral end of the clavicle and the scapula, and the scapulothoracic joint. The scapulothoracic joint is not a traditional joint in the sense of bone articulating directly with bone (see **joint classification**). Instead, the flattened scapula can glide over the posterior aspect of the thoracic cage. The scapula can elevate (move up), depress (move down), upwardly and downwardly rotate, retract (adduct), and protract (abduct) on the thorax. As a result of these movements, the position of the glenoid fossa of the scapula is altered and, as a consequence, the glenohumeral joint is moved. This arrangement enables a greater range of motion at the shoulder than would be possible by movement of the glenohumeral joint alone. The interaction between the scapulothoracic and glenohumeral joints is known as 'scapulohumeral rhythm'.

The shoulder is one of the most commonly injured sites in swimmers. Because their body weight is supported and the sport is a non-contact one, swimmers do not tend to suffer from traumatic injuries. However, overuse injuries are common, owing mainly to the stereotyped repetition of movements and large training loads of competitive swimmers. Because of the large range of shoulder motion required by the arm action in swimming, an injury known as 'swimmer's shoulder' or subacromial impingement syndrome may occur (see **In Sports 5**). This is inflammation of the tendon of supraspinatus, a shoulder muscle responsible for abducting the arm, secondary to it being pinched under the acromion process of the scapula.

Dislocation of the glenohumeral joint is a common acute shoulder injury associated with contact team sports, such as rugby and American football. Shoulder dislocation is also common in individual contact sports such as judo and wrestling. The mechanism of injury is typically a fall onto an abducted and externally rotated arm. The other common acute injury at the shoulder is damage to the acromioclavicular ligaments, or a 'separated shoulder'. Falling on the outstretched arm or directly onto the point of the shoulder can result in damage to these ligaments, producing a noticeable step at the lateral end of the clavicle; the size of the step depends on the extent of disruption of the acromioclavicular ligaments and the adjacent coracoclavicular ligaments (see **shoulder complex – ligaments**).

Further Reading

Struyf, F., Tate, A., Kuppens, K., Feijen, S., & Michener, L. A. (2017). Musculoskeletal dysfunctions associated with swimmers' shoulder. *British Journal of Sports Medicine, 51*, 775–780. doi: 10.1136/bjsports-2016-096847.

See also: **shoulder complex; shoulder complex – bones; shoulder complex – muscles; thoracic region.**

In Sports 5 Subacromial Impingement Syndrome

Subacromial impingement syndrome is an overuse injury of the shoulder complex that is common in swimmers. The injury causes pain at the shoulder in the region of the acromion process and is attributed to the irritation of soft tissue by repeated compression where it lies within the subacromial space. The name 'subacromial impingement syndrome' describes the location of the injury – below the acromion (subacromial) – and the type of damage – touching and compressing the soft tissue (impingement). The subacromial space is between the acromion process and the head of the humerus. Certain positions of the humerus relative to the acromion can reduce the size of the subacromial space and lead to tissue impingement. In particular, abduction and internal rotation of the humerus relative to the scapula both reduce the subacromial space, with the largest effect when both positions are combined. Scapulohumeral rhythm, which is the coordinated movement of the scapula with the humerus, helps to minimize the reduction in the subacromial space during daily movements. However, at extreme ranges of motion or when scapulohumeral rhythm is disrupted, this protective effect is lost. The tissue which is compressed and damaged by subacromial impingement is the supraspinatus muscle, which is the most superior of the muscles of the rotator cuff. Supraspinatus passes directly between the acromion and the head of the humerus, right through the subacromial space. This injury is common in swimmers due to the high repetitions, high loads, and extreme positions at the shoulder during the swimming strokes, particularly freestyle. Swimmers traditionally swim very high volumes with many thousands of shoulder revolutions, predisposing them to overuse injury of the shoulder. As with all overuse injuries, small deviations in technique or coordination may have a large effect when multiplied by the high number of repetitions completed during training. The direct cause of subacromial impingement in swimmers is unclear as no research studies have followed swimmers from the start of their swimming career to see what characteristics lead to injury down the road. Several deficits have been linked to subacromial impingement, but they may be a result of the injury and not the cause. These deficits include reduced shoulder, rotator cuff, and core muscle endurance, joint laxity (excessive flexibility and range of motion), and errors in swimming technique. As with all overuse injuries, the pain will decrease with rest that allows the damaged tissues to heal, but the injury will likely recur once swimming is restarted if the underlying causes are not addressed.

Further Reading

Struyf, F., Tate, A., Kuppens, K., Feijen, S., & Michener, L.A. (2017). Musculoskeletal dysfunctions associated with swimmers' shoulder. *British Journal of Sports Medicine, 51*, 775–780. doi: 10.1136/bjsports-2016-096847.

Shoulder Complex – Ligaments

The synovial joints of the shoulder complex are the glenohumeral and acromioclavicular joints. The scapulothoracic articulation is not a traditional joint and does not have ligaments associated with it. The glenohumeral joint is the primary joint of the shoulder, between the trunk and upper extremity. This joint is a shallow ball and socket joint which relies on its soft tissue structures for stability and support (Figure 20). The ligaments of the glenohumeral joint are thickenings of the joint capsule. They are the glenohumeral ligament and the coracohumeral ligament. The glenohumeral ligament is an anterior thickening of the joint capsule. It consists of superior, middle and inferior parts. It is not particularly strong and is vulnerable to damage during traumatic injuries, such as glenohumeral joint dislocation (see **shoulder complex – joints**). The coracohumeral ligament runs from the coracoid process of the scapula to the greater and lesser tubercles of the humerus. It is a superior thickening of the joint capsule. This strong ligament helps to support the weight of the upper limb which hangs from the glenoid fossa. Due to its lack of bony support and limited contribution from the glenohumeral ligament, the glenohumeral joint relies heavily on the muscles of the shoulder joint for support.

The acromioclavicular joint is also considered part of the shoulder girdle, since the acromion process is part of the scapula. Several ligaments connect the clavicle to the scapula. At this joint, the acromioclavicular ligament is a thickening of the joint capsule, equivalent to the glenohumeral ligament at the glenohumeral joint. In addition, coracoclavicular ligaments, between the coracoid process and the clavicle assist in keeping the clavicle in place. These ligaments attach to the clavicle medial to the acromioclavicular joint and connect to the coracoid process inferiorly. There are two distinct coracoclavicular ligaments, the trapezoid and conoid, named according to their shape (trapezoidal and cone-shaped). The conoid is the more medial of the two. The important role of these ligaments becomes apparent after an acromioclavicular joint separation. This injury is a dislocation of the acromioclavicular joint which typically occurs as a result of a fall directly onto the shoulder. The severity of the injury is determined by the degree of separation of the clavicle from the acromion process. If only the acromioclavicular joint is torn, there is no apparent separation of the joint because the coracoclavicular ligaments keep the clavicle in place. In a more severe injury, the coracoclavicular

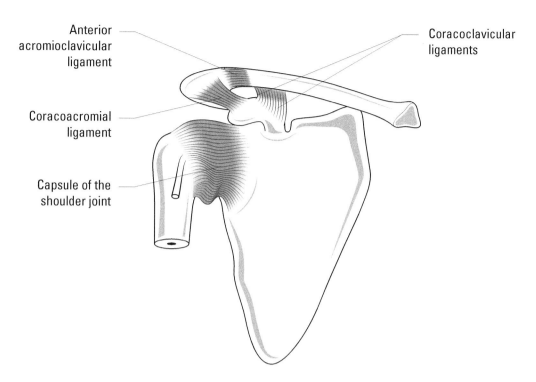

Anterior
acromioclavicular
ligament

Coracoclavicular
ligaments

Coracoacromial
ligament

Capsule of the
shoulder joint

Figure 20 Ligaments of the right shoulder. Adapted from Watkins (2014).

ligaments are also torn, and the clavicle is now free to move superiorly and become separated from the acromion. In this case, the lateral end of the clavicle can be identified clearly under the skin as a bump on the superior aspect of the shoulder.

See also: **shoulder complex; shoulder complex – bones; shoulder complex – joints; shoulder complex – ligaments; shoulder complex – muscles; thoracic region.**

Shoulder Complex – Muscles

The muscles of the shoulder are responsible for the multiaxial rotations that occur at the glenohumeral joint, as well as dynamic stabilization of the joint during activity (Figure 21; Table 7). Muscular stabilization helps to prevent dislocation of the head of the humerus from its shallow socket in the glenoid fossa of the scapula. The muscles of the glenohumeral joint are deltoid, pectoralis major, coracobrachialis, latissimus dorsi, teres major, and the four rotator cuff muscles. The muscles of the rotator cuff are subscapularis, supraspinatus, infraspinatus, and teres minor. The muscles of the scapulothoracic joint are trapezius, rhomboid major and minor, levator scapula, pectoralis minor, and serratus anterior.

The most superficial muscle of the shoulder is the deltoid, which has anterior, middle, and posterior heads and gives the shoulder its characteristic rounded shape. As a whole, the deltoid abducts the arm. The anterior deltoid flexes and internally rotates the arm and the posterior deltoid extends and externally rotates the arm. Pectoralis major flexes and internally rotates the arm from its anatomical reference position. The muscle is a powerful horizontal adductor of the arm and an extensor of the arm from a vertical position. The latissimus dorsi extends, adducts, and internally rotates the arm. Teres major adducts and extends the arm and contributes to internal rotation. Coracobrachialis helps to flex and adduct the arm.

The glenohumeral joint relies heavily on its soft tissues to stabilize it because the glenoid fossa of the scapula provides only a shallow socket in which the head of the humerus sits (see **shoulder complex – joints**). Stability of the joint is achieved passively by the ligaments that span the joint and functionally by the muscles surrounding the joint. Muscles are responsible for both joint rotation movements and drawing the bones together to strengthen the joint and maintain its integrity. The major role of the infraspinatus, supraspinatus, subscapularis, and teres minor muscles – the rotator cuff – is strengthening and stabilizing the shoulder joint

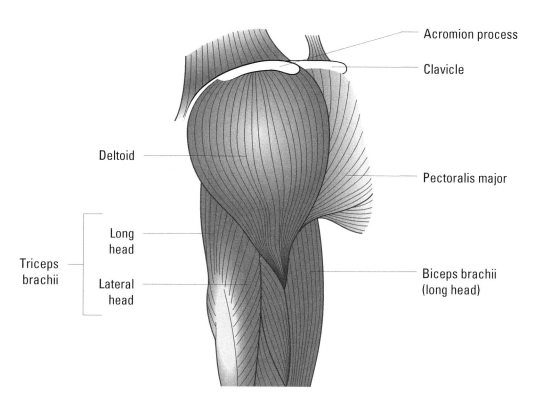

Figure 21 Muscles of the right shoulder

Table 7 Shoulder muscles contributing to joint movements

Joint movement	Muscles
Glenohumeral joint	
Shoulder flexion	Pectoralis major (from anatomical position), anterior deltoid, biceps brachii, coracobrachialis
Shoulder extension	Latissimus dorsi, posterior deltoid, teres major, pectoralis major (from vertical position)
Shoulder adduction	Latissimus dorsi, pectoralis major, teres major, subscapularis, coracobrachialis
Shoulder abduction	Deltoid, supraspinatus
Shoulder internal rotation	Pectoralis major, latissimus dorsi, anterior deltoid, teres major, subscapularis
Shoulder external rotation	Posterior deltoid, infraspinatus, teres minor
Shoulder horizontal adduction	Pectoralis major, anterior deltoid
Shoulder horizontal abduction	Posterior deltoid, infraspinatus, teres minor
Scapulothoracic joint	
Scapula elevation	Trapezius (upper portion), levator scapula
Scapula depression	Trapezius (lower portion), pectoralis major, pectoralis minor
Scapula protraction	Serratus anterior
Scapula retraction	Trapezius (middle portion), rhomboid major, rhomboid minor
Scapula upward rotation	Trapezius (upper portion)
Scapular downward rotation	Levator scapula

The rotator cuff consists of subscapularis, supraspinatus, infraspinatus, and teres minor.

by drawing the humerus into the glenoid fossa. The glenoid fossa is shallow and almost vertical in orientation, therefore, the supraspinatus plays a major role in preventing downward dislocation of the humerus when carrying heavy weights in the hand. The infraspinatus and teres minor muscles also play a role in externally rotating the arm. Subscapularis internally rotates the arm and supraspinatus abducts the arm.

The scapula moves on the back of the thorax at the scapulothoracic joint. The large trapezius muscle contributes to several movements of the scapula, depending on which part is contracting. The upper part of trapezius elevates the scapula along with levator scapula. The lower part of trapezius depresses the scapula. Serratus anterior is responsible for protracting the scapula and the middle part of trapezius and the rhomboids retract the scapula. The upper part of trapezius upwardly rotates the scapula while levator scapula moves the scapula in downward rotation.

The muscles of the shoulder region can be strengthened primarily by various dumbbell exercises, which recruit different parts of the muscles depending on whether the dumbbell is raised to the front, side, or rear of the body. Dumbbell raises are single joint exercises that isolate the movements of the shoulder. The shoulder muscles are also recruited in compound exercises that mainly involve the large chest or back muscles, such as bench press and rowing exercises respectively. In these exercises, which more closely mimic the likely role of the shoulder during activity, the shoulder muscles contribute to abduction, adduction, flexion, extension, horizontal abduction, and horizontal adduction at the shoulder, as well as providing stability of the shoulder joint and a strong link between the arms and the trunk. The dual role of the shoulder muscles in joint rotation and stability is well illustrated by the role of the shoulder in rowing. For a large part of the drive phase, the shoulder muscles are responsible for shoulder joint stability and the effective transfer of power from the lower body to the oar in the hands of the rower. However, at the end of the stroke, the shoulder muscles act concentrically in extending and then flexing the shoulder as the oar is removed from the water at the end of the stroke.

See also: **muscle; shoulder complex; shoulder complex – bones; shoulder complex – joints; shoulder complex – ligaments; thoracic region.**

Thoracic Region

The thoracic spine consists of 12 vertebrae and is less mobile than the flexible cervical spine above it (see **head and neck – bones**). There are 12 pairs of ribs in the thoracic cage. Each thoracic vertebra articulates with one or two pairs of ribs and the ribs are attached to the sternum anteriorly. As a result of participating in sports activities that require the thoracic spine to be held in a single position for long periods, the intervertebral joints can become stiff and the thoracic spine immobile. This can result in overload of the more flexible cervical spine, which becomes hypermobile to enable the head to maintain its position with respect to the rest of the body. In this situation, the spinal processes of the cervical vertebrae can become inflamed and painful to the touch.

See also: thoracic region – bones; thoracic region – joints; thoracic region – ligaments; thoracic region – muscles.

Thoracic Region – Bones

The bones of the thoracic (chest) region are the thoracic vertebrae, sternum, clavicle, and ribs (Figure 22). The costal cartilages are also integral to the structure of this region. This region contains the heart and the lungs, around which the bones of the thorax form a protective cage. There are 12 thoracic vertebrae, each of which has two associated ribs. The 10 superior pairs, seven pairs of true and three pairs of false ribs, are each attached to the sternum (breastbone) anteriorly by the costal cartilage. The first seven pairs of ribs articulate with the sternum directly via their own costal cartilage and are true ribs. The remaining three pairs of anteriorly secured ribs articulate only indirectly with the sternum via the costal cartilage of the rib above. The last two pairs are the floating (free) ribs, which do not have an anterior attachment and are attached only to the eleventh and twelfth lumbar vertebrae respectively. The sternum is divided into three parts. The manubrium is the most superior part and articulates with the first and second pairs of ribs and the clavicle. The body is the largest piece and articulates with the second to seventh pairs of ribs. The most distal part is the xiphoid process, which does not articulate with the ribs.

The basic structure of a rib consists of two ends and a flattened body or shaft. The vertebral end is known as the head and articulates with the body of a thoracic

(a) Anterior view

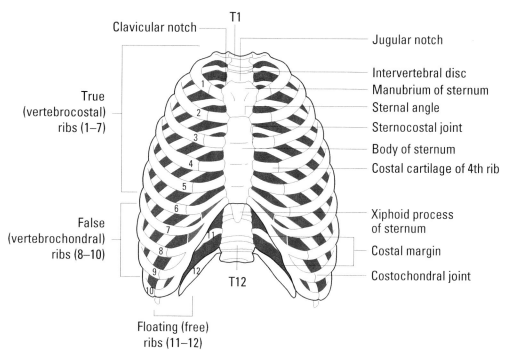

(b) Posterior view

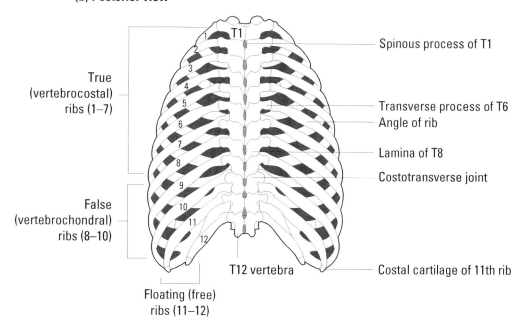

Figure 22 Bones of the thoracic region

vertebra. The rib tubercle, located anterior to the neck of the rib, has an articular facet that articulates with the vertebral transverse process. The anterior end of the rib articulates with the sternum via its own costal cartilage (true ribs), or indirectly via the costal cartilage of the rib above (false ribs). The floating ribs do not articulate with any bony structure anteriorly. The ribs increase in length from the first to the seventh; their length then decreases from the seventh to the twelfth. The body of the rib is grooved where the intercostal muscles of the thorax attach. Ribs are highly vascularized bones and consist mainly of cancellous bone inside a thin layer of compact **bone**. The first and second pairs of ribs are somewhat different in structure that the third through tenth pairs. The flattened body of the first two pairs is oriented transversely, whereas the remaining pairs are oriented vertically. The angle (curve) of the first two pairs is also much sharper. The floating ribs also differ in structure from the typical ribs because they are much shorter, almost straight and do not articulate with the transverse processes of the thoracic vertebrae.

Athletes who participate in contact sports are at risk of traumatic injury to the ribs. Although painful, these injuries are rarely serious and heal rapidly because the bone is highly vascularized. Overuse injuries can also occur in the thoracic region. This type of injury may occur when the thoracic region is under tension and forms a rigid link between the upper and lower body for the transfer of load. For example, rib stress fractures are relatively common in competitive rowers and are thought to be related to the forces transmitted through the body from the feet pushing against the foot stretcher of the boat to the oar in the hands.

See also: **bone; bone classification; core stability; thoracic region; thoracic region – joints; thoracic region – ligaments; thoracic region – muscles.**

Thoracic Region – Joints

The thoracic region consists of the thoracic spine, ribs, and sternum. The joints of this region are the sternoclavicular joint, the intervertebral joints, and the anterior and posterior articulations of the ribs. The thoracic spine is less mobile than the cervical spine, despite having more (12) vertebrae than the cervical spine (7). The sternoclavicular joint is formed between the sternal end of the clavicle and the clavicular notch of the manubrium of the sternum.

The intervertebral articulations of the thoracic spine are those between the vertebral bodies and those between the vertebral arches. These joints allow only small movements between adjacent vertebrae. However, when these small movements are summed across the whole of the thoracic spine, they add up to significant flexion and extension of the region as a whole. The articulations between the vertebral bodies are symphyses (see **joint classification**). The intervertebral discs are the main connection between adjacent vertebrae. These flexible discs of fibrous tissue and fibrocartilage act as shock absorbers for the spine as a whole and attenuate forces travelling up the body to protect the brain from exposure to excessive shock. The articulations between the inferior and superior articular processes on the vertebral arches are synovial gliding joints. The anterior and posterior longitudinal ligaments are associated with these articulations, as well as the intervertebral discs. The thoracic vertebral arches are connected by the following restraining ligaments: ligamentum flavum, supraspinous ligament, and interspinous ligament.

Joints found only in the thoracic region of the vertebral column are the costovertebral and costotransverse joints. These are the articulations between the thoracic vertebrae and ribs. The costovertebral joint is between the vertebral body (see **vertebral structure**) and the head of the rib. The costotransverse joint is between the transverse process of the vertebra and the articular facet of the rib tubercle. Most ribs articulate with two adjacent vertebral bodies and the costotransverse joint is formed with the transverse process of the inferior vertebrae.

The spinal column can move in flexion, extension, lateral flexion, axial rotation, and circumduction. Overall, the largest movement is flexion, followed by extension, lateral flexion, and rotation. Only a little circumduction is possible in the spine. These movements are reduced in the thoracic region compared to the cervical region to prevent them interfering with breathing. The most significant movement in the thoracic region is axial rotation (see **planes and axes of movement**). Flexion and extension are reduced by the articular processes of the vertebrae being directed anteriorly and posteriorly; lateral flexion is restricted by the presence of the ribs and sternum.

The cartilaginous joints between the anterior part of the ribs and the sternum are a weak point that is subject to dislocation injury. In sporting activities in which the trunk acts as a rigid link between the upper and lower body for the transfer of power, the joints of the thoracic region are under considerable tension. This occurs in rowing, and rowers are susceptible to instances of the tip of a rib being dislocated or 'popping out' of its anterior articulation with the sternum. A similar injury can occur with the simple act of coughing. Again, the tension generated in the torso results in one of the ribs becoming dislocated anteriorly. This injury is particularly painful while breathing in and is easily localized to the dislocated rib. Typical treatment for this injury is physiotherapy that mobilizes this region and actively pushes the displaced rib back into the correct position. Relocation of the rib provides an immediate reduction in pain and is key to having a thorax that is stable under tension.

See also: **thoracic region; thoracic region – bones; thoracic region – ligaments; thoracic region – muscles.**

Thoracic Region – Ligaments

The thoracic region contains many joints, and each has several ligaments associated with it. In the thoracic spine are the intervertebral, costovertebral and costotransverse joints. The vertebral column has several ligaments which run its whole length, connecting all of the vertebrae together, either as one continuous long ligament or a series of shorter ligaments found between each adjacent pair of vertebrae. From anterior to posterior these are the anterior longitudinal ligament, the posterior longitudinal ligament, the ligamentum flavum, the interspinous ligaments, and the supraspinous ligament.

The anterior longitudinal ligament is wide and strong. It runs along the anterior side of the vertebral bodies and attaches to both the vertebrae and intervertebral discs. It helps to prevent hyperextension of the back. The posterior longitudinal is narrower and weaker than the anterior ligament. It runs along the posterior side of the vertebral bodies, inside the vertebral canal (see **vertebral structure**). This ligament attaches only to the intervertebral discs and its role is to help prevent hyperflexion of the spine. The ligamentum flava are a series of ligaments which join the laminae of adjacent vertebral arches together, making up the posterior wall of the vertebral canal. They derive their name from its unusual yellow colour ('flavum' in Latin), which is due to their high elastin content. Ligaments are usually inextensible cords, but the ligamentum flavum is more like an elastic band. It stretches when the trunk flexes, which helps to prevent rapid flexion that might result in injury to the intervertebral discs. It then recoils as the trunk extends and assists with this movement. The interspinous ligaments link the bodies of adjacent spinous processes throughout the vertebral column, and are relatively weak. The supraspinous ligament connects the tips of the spinous processes and is much stronger, helping to prevent hyperflexion of the back. Additional, smaller ligaments include the intertransverse ligaments, which link adjacent transverse processes. These are stronger in the thoracic region than elsewhere in the vertebral column.

There are two types of joint between the ribs and the vertebrae in the thoracic region: the costovertebral and costotransverse joints. The costovertebral joint is between the head of the rib and the vertebral body. The radiate ligament crosses this joint. The ligament is so-named because it fans out from the head of the rib to its insertions on the vertebral body. The costotransverse joint is between the tubercle of the rib and the transverse process of the vertebra. There are lateral and superior costotransverse ligaments at this joint. The lateral costotransverse ligament passes from the rib tubercle to the transverse process it articulates with. The superior costotransverse ligament passes from the superior border of the rib to the transverse process of the vertebra above.

The sternoclavicular joint, between the sternum of the thoracic cage and the clavicle, has several ligaments associated with it. There are anterior and posterior sternoclavicular ligaments which pass directly across the joint. In addition, there is an interclavicular ligament which passes between the right and left clavicles, across the suprasternal notch. There is also a costoclavicular ligament lateral to the joint. This ligament passes from the first rib to the clavicle and assists in keeping the medial end of the clavicle in place.

See also: **shoulder complex – joints; thoracic region; thoracic region – bones; thoracic region – joints; thoracic region – muscles.**

Thoracic Region – Muscles

The muscles of the thorax often play dual roles, generating movement in the thorax and shoulder through concentric contraction (see **muscle contraction – types**) and stabilizing the upper body through eccentric or isometric contraction. The muscles of this region are at risk of traumatic injury, in the form of muscle strains and tears sustained during ballistic activities, and overuse injury that often results from imbalances in muscular development.

The muscles that connect the upper limb to the vertebral column are trapezius, latissimus dorsi, the major and minor rhomboids and the levator scapulae (see shoulder complex – muscles). The trapezius also contributes to extending the neck (see **head and neck – muscles**). The muscles that connect the upper limb to the anterior and lateral thorax are pectoralis major and minor, and serratus anterior (Figure 23; Table 8).

The muscles of the thorax itself are the internal and external intercostals, subcostals, transverse thoracis, levatores costarum, inferior and superior serratus posterior, and the diaphragm. The 11 intercostal muscles lie between the ribs and draw adjacent ribs together. When the first rib is braced by the scalene muscles that run between it and the cervical vertebrae, the external intercostals increase the volume of the thoracic cavity by raising the ribs on contraction. Conversely, when the last rib is braced by the quadratus lumborum muscle in the lumbar region, the internal intercostals decrease the volume of the thoracic cavity. Similarly, the action of transversus thoracis is to draw the anterior part of the ribs distally and decrease the volume of the thoracic cavity. The levatores costarum and superior serratus posterior raise the ribs and increase the thoracic volume. The inferior serratus posterior draws the distal ribs outwards and downwards, counteracting the inward pull of the diaphragm.

The diaphragm is a musculofibrous sheet that separates the thoracic cavity, containing the lungs and the heart, from the abdominal cavity. The diaphragm plays a key role in breathing because it changes the volume and pressure in the thoracic cavity as it moves. During inhalation, the diaphragm lowers and flattens, increasing the volume and decreasing the pressure within the thoracic cavity. Consequently, the ambient air pressure outside the body is higher than that within the thorax, and air is forced into the lungs. During exhalation, the opposite occurs and the decrease in volume and increase in pressure within the thorax force air out of the lungs.

The deep muscles of the back as a whole extend the trunk (Figure 24). This group includes the erector spinae, the splenius, semispinalis, multifidus, interspinales, and intertransversarii. These deep spinal muscles are also involved in stabilizing the trunk, particularly multifidus, which works in conjunction with the transverse abdominals to stabilize the lumbar region (see **Hot Topic 4**).

The thoracic region is subject to both traumatic and overuse injuries. Traumatic muscle strains and tears occur in sports, such as squash, which demand rapid movements of the torso and frequently place the spine in twisted and hyperextended positions.

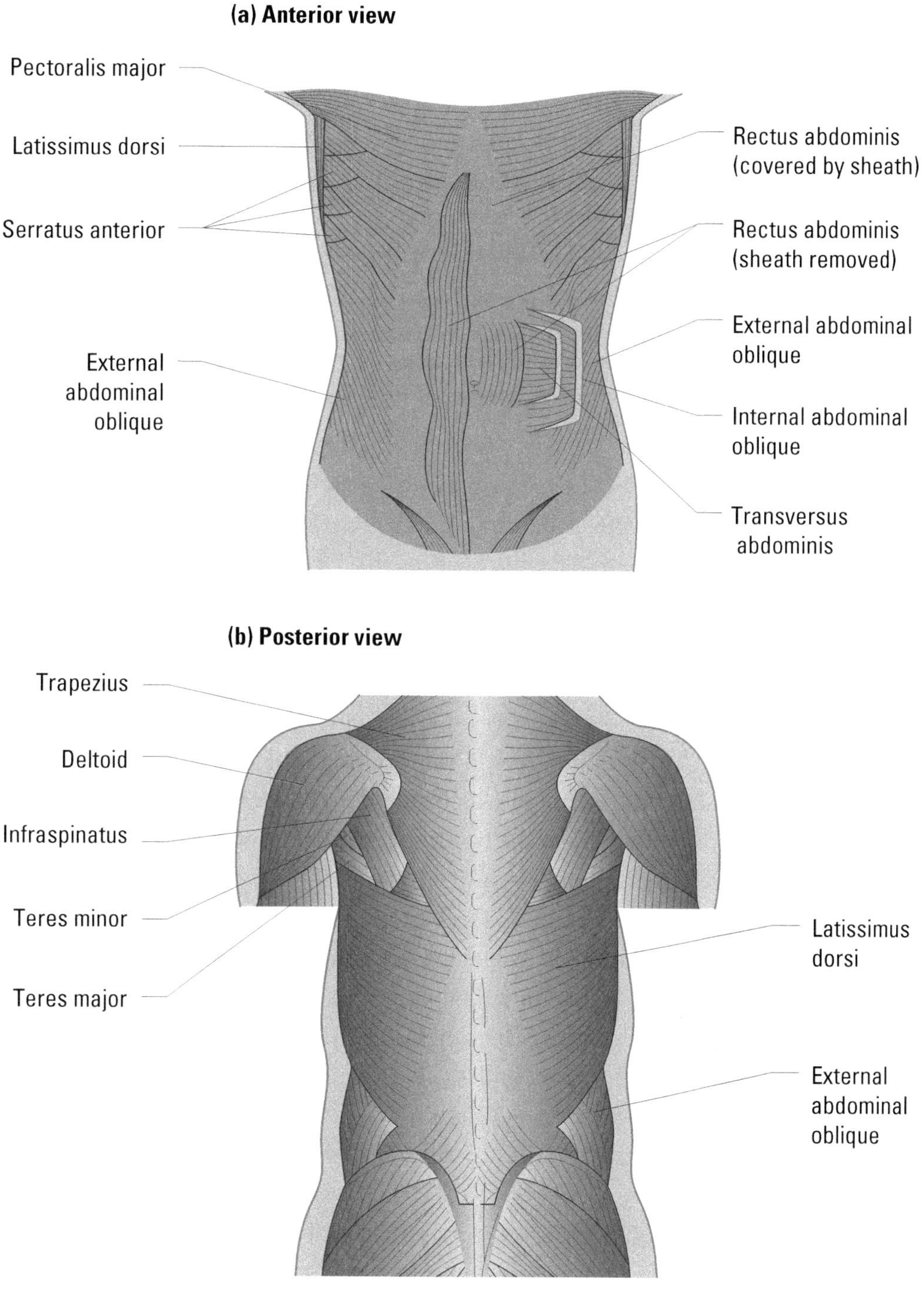

(a) Anterior view

Pectoralis major

Latissimus dorsi

Serratus anterior

External
abdominal
oblique

Rectus abdominis
(covered by sheath)

Rectus abdominis
(sheath removed)

External abdominal
oblique

Internal abdominal
oblique

Transversus
abdominis

(b) Posterior view

Trapezius

Deltoid

Infraspinatus

Teres minor

Teres major

Latissimus
dorsi

External
abdominal
oblique

Figure 23 Superficial muscles of the thoracic region. Adapted from Sewell et al. (2013).

Table 8 Thorax muscles contributing to joint movements

Joint movement	Muscles
Trunk flexion	Both*: rectus abdominis, internal obliques, external obliques
Trunk extension	Both*: iliocostalis, longissimus, spinalis
Lateral flexion to the right**	Right: iliocostalis, longissimus, spinalis, external oblique, internal oblique
Rotation to the right**	Right internal oblique, left external oblique

Notes: * Both indicates this is the action when both muscles contract together.

** A direction is given for lateral flexion and rotation to illustrate whether the individual muscle on the same or opposite side to the direction of movement is active.

The erector spinae consists of iliocostalis, longissimus, and spinalis.

Activities that involve one side of the body more than the other have the potential to create muscular imbalances that may lead to more serious bony misalignment problems if they are allowed to persist unchecked. For example, sweep oar rowing, in which the rower has only one oar, emphasizes twisting and leaning of the trunk towards the side that the oar is on. Since rowing is an activity that requires much strength and muscular development in the trunk, this can lead to the development of strength imbalances and asymmetries. Eventually, these muscular imbalances can lead to skeletal changes and introduce scoliosis into the spine of the rower, such that it is possible to determine which side the athlete rows on by looking at the inclination of the shoulders in the frontal plane. The rowing action encourages the shoulder nearest to the oar to be held lower than the outside shoulder to enable a longer stroke to be obtained. The best prevention against the development of these structural imbalances is to ensure that supplementary training, such as weight lifting, focuses on the symmetrical development of strength on both sides of the body. Similarly, flexibility programmes should be designed to ensure that flexibility of the shoulders, trunk, and the lower extremities is symmetrical, and that any muscle shortening that develops as a result of the rowing technique is counteracted by actively working to stretch and lengthen the muscle groups involved.

There are many weight-lifting exercises that will strengthen the muscles of the thoracic region; these can be divided into single joint isolation exercises and compound exercises. In general, compound exercises reflect the action of muscles during sports activities more closely, since it is quite unusual for an activity to

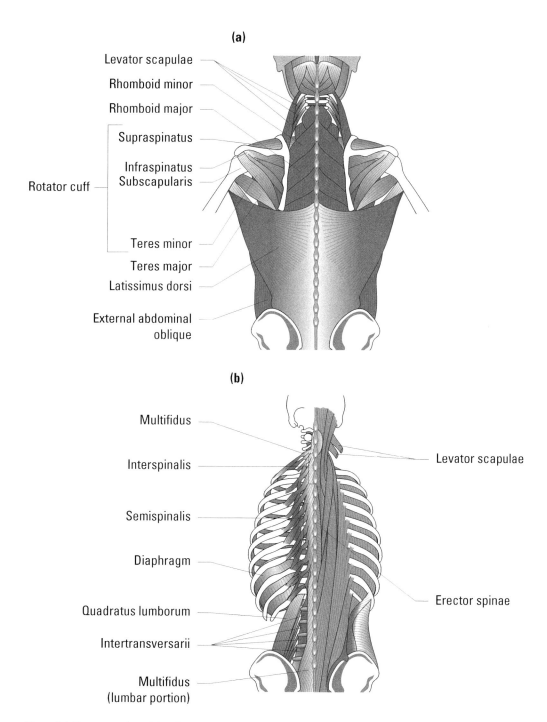

Figure 24 Deep muscles of the thoracic region (including muscles of the head and neck and lumbar spine and pelvis). Adapted from Sewell et al. (2013).

involve movement only at a single joint. Examples of compound exercises for the muscles of the thorax include chest presses and back rows. Chest presses of all types develop the pectoralis major mainly and also parts of the deltoid and the triceps, which are involved in movement and stabilization of the upper extremity. Back rows develop the latissimus dorsi, plus the trapezius, rhomboids, and parts of the deltoid and the biceps brachii that are involved in stabilization of the scapula and movement of the arms during the exercise.

See also: **muscle; shoulder complex – muscles; thoracic region; thoracic region – bones; thoracic region – joints; thoracic region – ligaments.**

Vertebral Structure

There are 33 vertebrae in the human spine, divided into four regions. From the base of the skull down, these are the 7 cervical vertebrae of the neck, 12 thoracic vertebrae of the upper and middle back, 5 lumbar vertebrae in the lower back, and the fused vertebrae of the pelvic region. There are 5 fused vertebrae in the sacrum and 4 in the coccyx. The vertebrae within a section are numbered in a superior to inferior direction.

The basic structure of the 24 moveable vertebrae is similar (Figure 25). The main body of a vertebra is roughly cylindrical and oriented anteriorly, in front of the spinal cord. Immediately posterior to the body is a hole (vertebral foramen), through which the spinal cord passes down the entire length of the vertebral column. The bony structure surrounding the vertebral canal is known as the vertebral, or neural, arch. The parts of the arch that attach directly to the vertebral body are the two pedicles. The parts that surround the canal laterally and dorsally are the two laminae. Each vertebra has 7 processes, 4 that articulate with adjacent vertebrae and 3 for muscular attachment. Each lamina has a superior and an inferior articular process, plus a transverse process for the attachment of muscles and ligaments. Each vertebra has a dorsally projecting spinous process.

The vertebrae of the different regions of the spine have slight variations from this basic structure. The cervical vertebrae are the smallest of the independently moveable vertebrae and can easily be distinguished by the presence of an additional hole (transverse foramen) in each of the transverse processes. Several of them have interesting deviations from the basic structure described above. The first cervical vertebra is known as the atlas and has a ring-like structure without a defined vertebral body. The second cervical vertebra is called the axis because the atlas and the head rotate on it, around the superiorly projecting dens of the axis. The final, seventh, cervical vertebra has a long spinous process that can be palpated easily.

Thoracic vertebrae are the only ones with costal facets on the body and transverse processes for articulation with the ribs (see **thoracic region – joints**). Additionally, the orientation of the superior and inferior articular processes differs between the regions. In the thoracic region, the articular processes face posteriorly (superior processes) and anteriorly (inferior processes). This arrangement prevents flexion and extension from occurring in this region, but allows axial rotation. Lateral flexion is also possible, but is limited by the thoracic cage (see **thoracic region – bones**). In the lumbar vertebrae, the articular processes face posteromedially (superior) and anterolaterally (inferior). This provides rotational stability and allows flexion and extension to occur between adjacent vertebrae.

The size of the vertebrae increases down the spine, with the largest individual vertebrae being found in the lumbar spine. Overuse stress fractures can occur in the lumbar spine of cricket bowlers. This common injury, known as spondylolysis, is one of the few overuse injuries in sport that have been shown to have a statistically significant relationship to a particular technique. This injury is predominantly found in bowlers who use the mixed technique; this is a hybrid technique with aspects of both of the two traditional bowling techniques – front-on and side-on. The combination of a front-on lower body and a side-on upper body position during the delivery stride, when the forces being transmitted up the standing leg may be up to six times the body weight, places the lumbar spine in a twisted, hyperextended, laterally flexed, and axially-loaded position. Elucidation of this significant relationship has led to the mixed technique being actively discouraged in young bowlers.

Further Reading

Morton, S., Barton, C. J., Rice, S. & Morrissey, D. (2014). Risk factors and successful interventions for cricket-related low back pain: A systematic review. *British Journal of Sports Medicine, 48*, 685–691.

See also: **axial skeleton; head and neck – bones; lumbar spine and pelvis – bones; thoracic region – bones.**

(a) Superior view

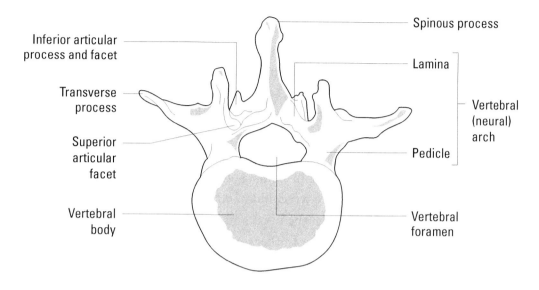

Spinous process

Inferior articular process and facet

Lamina

Transverse process

Vertebral (neural) arch

Superior articular facet

Pedicle

Vertebral body

Vertebral foramen

(b) Lateral view

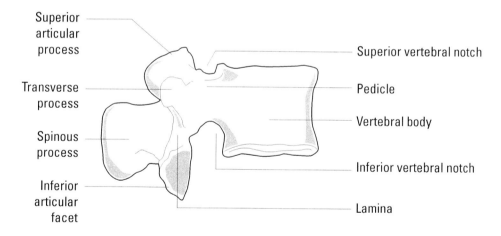

Superior articular process

Superior vertebral notch

Transverse process

Pedicle

Vertebral body

Spinous process

Inferior vertebral notch

Inferior articular facet

Lamina

Figure 25 Structure of a typical vertebra

Wrist and Hand

The wrist and hand complex has many joints, which provide flexibility and enable the hand to grasp and manipulate objects in the world around us. The many bones and joints in the hand enable it to perform multiple tasks during various activities. Each of the digits can operate independently, for example, when playing a musical instrument, or the hand can make use of the opposable thumb to encircle and hold various implements. Furthermore, owing to the flexibility of the shoulder joint (see **shoulder complex – joints**) and the **elbow and forearm – joints**, the position of the hand relative to the body can be finely controlled.

When they are the main point of contact with equipment, the opponent, or the ground in sport activities, the wrist and hand are at risk of injury. Depending on the forces transmitted through the wrist and hand, and the frequency of force repetition, the athlete can be at risk of either traumatic or overuse injury. Traumatic injuries in this region include fracture of the scaphoid, the largest carpal bone, and the individual phalanges of the digits. Overuse injuries include cyclist's palsy, a neuropathy related to excessive pressure on the ulnar nerve at the wrist (see **wrist and hand – joints**).

See also: wrist and hand – bones; wrist and hand – joints; wrist and hand – ligaments; wrist and hand – muscles.

Wrist and Hand – Bones

The wrist and hand contain many bones and joints, giving the region high flexibility. The hand is the major point of contact between the body and objects in the surrounding world; the flexibility of this region enables an individual to adapt easily to different holding and gripping requirements. The wrist and hand are also strong enough to support the entire body in sports such as gymnastics. The proximal bones of the wrist are the radius and ulna of the forearm (see **elbow and forearm – bones**). The eight carpal bones are the scaphoid, lunate, triquetral, pisiform, trapezium, trapezoid, capitate, and hamate. These bones are arranged in two rows; the first four are more proximal and the last four more distal. The bones of the hand are the five metacarpals and the 14 phalanges of the digits – the thumb has two, whereas the fingers each have three (Figure 26).

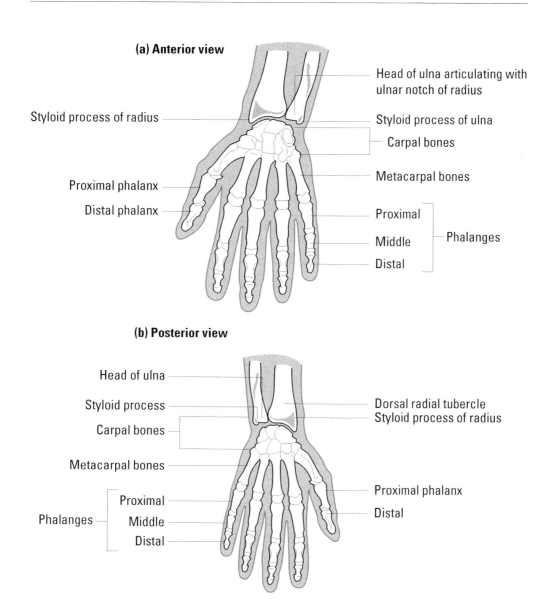

(a) Anterior view

Head of ulna articulating with ulnar notch of radius

Styloid process of radius

Styloid process of ulna

Carpal bones

Metacarpal bones

Proximal phalanx

Distal phalanx

Proximal

Middle — Phalanges

Distal

(b) Posterior view

Head of ulna

Styloid process

Carpal bones

Metacarpal bones

Proximal
Phalanges — Middle
Distal

Dorsal radial tubercle
Styloid process of radius

Proximal phalanx

Distal

Figure 26 Bones of the right wrist and hand

The metacarpals of the hand are equivalent to the metatarsals of the foot (see **ankle and foot – bones**). They are long slender bones with a body and two articulating ends. The first metacarpal is that of the thumb and it articulates with the trapezium of the wrist. The second metacarpal articulates with the trapezium and the trapezoid as well as the third metacarpal. The third metacarpal articulates with the capitate of the wrist and the second and fourth metacarpals. The fourth metacarpal articulates with the third and fifth metacarpals, the capitate, and the hamate. The fifth metacarpal articulates with the fourth metacarpal and the hamate.

Although relatively uncommon, fracture of the scaphoid, the largest wrist bone, can occur as a result of a fall onto the outstretched hand. A fall of this nature can result in fracture of either the scaphoid or the radius, depending of the position of the wrist and hand at the moment of impact. Typically, if the wrist is fully extended, the scaphoid will fracture; lesser amounts of extension will likely result in fracture of the distal part of the radius. Acute fracture of the scaphoid may also occur as a result of striking an opponent in contact sports, such as rugby or American football, or in striking the ground or equipment with a hyperextended wrist in gymnastics. Although rare, this injury is potentially serious and may even be career-ending for the professional sports person as it has a high risk of complications.

See also: **bone; bone classification; wrist and hand – joints; wrist and hand – ligaments; wrist and hand – muscles.**

Wrist and Hand – Joints

The wrist and hand are a complex region containing many joints that provide flexibility and enable the hand to interact with its environment. This dexterity of the hand is essential because it provides direct interaction with the world around us and the objects in it. The major joint of this region is the radiocarpal (wrist) joint, the primary connection between the forearm and the hand. The bones of the carpal region have a little movement between them, mostly at the midcarpal joint between the proximal and distal rows of carpal bones. The intermetacarpal and carpometacarpal articulations give the palm of the hand its flexibility. The metacarpophalangeal joints – the knuckles – give the digits their independent movements and the interphalangeal joints enable the digits to flex and extend in grasping movements. Injuries of the wrist and hand can be both traumatic and overuse types.

The wrist is formed primarily between the distal end of the radius of the forearm and the carpal bones of the hand (radiocarpal joint) and indirectly with the ulna of the forearm (ulnocarpal joint); the ulna is separated from the carpal bones by an articular disc, although it is connected to them via ligaments. The carpal bones involved in the wrist joint are the scaphoid, lunate, and triquetral. These three bones together form a convex surface that articulates with the concave surface of the distal radius, forming a condyloid joint. The joint is supported by the palmar and dorsal radiocarpal and ulnar and radial collateral ligaments. The wrist is capable of flexion, extension, abduction, adduction, and circumduction movements. Extension is the largest movement occurring at the wrist, followed by flexion, then adduction, and abduction. Circumduction is achieved as a combination of these movements. No axial rotation is possible at the wrist; instead, this movement occurs through pronation and supination of the radius and ulna in the forearm (see **elbow and forearm – joints**).

The only carpometacarpal joint with any significant movement is that of the thumb – the first metacarpal. The movements permitted at this saddle joint are flexion and extension in the plane of the palm of the hand, abduction and adduction in a plane perpendicular to the palm of the hand, and opposition. The opposable thumb gives the hand its grasping ability by enabling the tip of the thumb to come into contact with the palmar surfaces of the fingers when they are slightly flexed. The ellipsoidal metacarpophalangeal joints, easily recognizable as the knuckles of the hand, also allow significant movement of the digits. This joint is capable of flexion and extension, abduction and adduction, and circumduction. Finally, the interphalangeal hinge joints of the fingers and thumb are capable of a large amount of flexion, enabling the hand to make a fist, and a little extension.

The wrist is prone to injury in a wide variety of sports. For example, the wrist is at risk of both traumatic and overuse injuries in gymnasts, as the upper limbs must often carry all of the body's weight in movements such as handsprings. Fractures and sprains of the wrist can occur when it is forced into hyperextension during a landing on the hands. Overuse injuries occur in gymnastics as a result of repetitive low-impact landings on the hands that do not load the joint sufficiently to cause an acute sprain or fracture, but instead cause microdamage that accumulates over time and eventually leads to injury as the damage accumulates faster than it can be repaired.

A common and potentially serious overuse injury that may occur in cyclists is 'cyclist's palsy', also known as ulnar neuropathy. This is a compression injury of the ulnar nerve at the wrist that causes tingling and numbness in the little finger and ring finger of the affected hand. If the injury is untreated and becomes more severe, it can lead to pain and weakness in the muscles of the hand and, eventually, coordination problems. If the injury is untreated, the coordination problems may become permanent. The cause of this injury is cycling for long periods with the hands flexed and a large proportion of the body weight resting on them, resulting in the ulnar nerve being compressed. This position is most severe when the hands are on the dropped part of the handlebars. As with most overuse injuries, correction of the source of the problem is essential to prevent the injury from returning after recovery and rehabilitation. When trying to identify the root cause of the injury, consideration should be given to the time spent in the dropped position on the handlebars, the padding in the gloves and on the handlebars, and the position of the cyclist on the bike. If the bike is too long for the rider or the handlebars are too low, this will result in the weight being thrown forwards on to the hands, increasing the loading at the wrist. Changes in bike set-up may be essential to position the cyclist more favourably on the bike.

See also: **wrist and hand; wrist and hand – bones; wrist and hand – ligaments; wrist and hand – muscles.**

Wrist and Hand – Ligaments

There are many bones in the wrist and hand, thus there are many joints and many ligaments associated with these joints. Within the hand, the basic pattern of ligaments is repeated across the digits, with some differences occurring at the thumb. Furthermore, while the wrist contains eight individual carpal bones that articulate with each other, the distal forearm and the proximal part of the hand, many of the ligaments restrain the wrist as a whole, rather than individual components.

There are several ligaments that limit movement of the wrist, in addition to the joint capsule. The posterior radiocarpal ligament runs diagonally across the posterior aspect of the wrist from the distal end of the radius to the triquetral and hamate carpal bones on the ulnar side of the wrist. This ligament limits flexion of the wrist. The anterior radiocarpal ligament runs from the anterior aspect of the distal end of the radius to the scaphoid, lunate and capitate bones of the wrist. This ligament limits extension of the wrist. The collateral ligaments of the wrist run along the sides of the joint to limit frontal plane motion. The ulnar collateral ligament, running from the styloid process of the ulna to the triquetral, limits abduction of the wrist. The radial collateral ligament, from the styloid process of the radius to the scaphoid bone, limits adduction of the wrist. Minimal movement occurs between the carpal bones themselves; they are held together by the anterior, posterior and interosseous carpal ligaments. The interlocking structure of the carpal bones also provides support for the wrist, in addition to the support provided by these ligaments.

Anterior to the carpal bones, superficial to the flexor tendons which cross the wrist, is the transverse carpal ligament (also known as the flexor retinaculum). This ligament forms the anterior wall of the carpal tunnel as it runs between the anterior prominences of the outer carpal bones on the radial and ulnar sides of the wrist.

Moving distally from the wrist to the fingertips, there are the following joints: carpometacarpal, intermetacarpal, metacarpophalangeal, and proximal and distal interphalangeal joints. Each joint has several ligaments associated with it. The carpometacarpal and intermetacarpal joints are supported by anterior, posterior and interosseous ligaments. The metacarpophalangeal joint (knuckle) has a more complex arrangement of ligaments. Anteriorly, strong palmar ligaments run from the distal end of the metacarpal to the proximal end of the proximal phalanx. Medial and lateral collateral ligaments also pass from the metacarpal to the phalanx. Additionally, the second to fifth metacarpal heads are linked together by deep transverse metacarpal ligaments. The arrangement of palmar and collateral ligaments is repeated at the interphalangeal joints of the digits.

See also: **wrist and hand; wrist and hand – bones; wrist and hand – joints; wrist and hand – muscles.**

Wrist and Hand – Muscles

The wrist and hand complex contains many joints, providing an individual with the flexibility to interact successfully with the environment. This dexterity is essential because the hand is the means of direct interaction with objects in the external world. The major joint of this region is the radiocarpal joint, the connection between the forearm and the hand. Additional joints in the palm, knuckles, and the digits give the hand its ability to move and grasp items (Table 9). The muscles of the wrist and extrinsic muscles of the hand are located in the forearm and described elsewhere (see **elbow and forearm – muscles**; see Figure 10). The intrinsic muscles are located within the hand itself and are considered here.

The muscles of the hand can be divided into three groups; those of the thumb (thenar muscles), the little finger (hypothenar muscles), and the palmar region

Table 9 Wrist and hand muscles contributing to joint movements

Joint movement	Muscles
Wrist flexion	Palmaris longus, flexor carpi radialis, flexor carpi ulnaris, flexor digitorum superficialis, flexor digitorum profundus
Wrist extension	Extensor carpi radialis longus, extensor carpi radialis brevis, extensor carpi ulnaris, extensor digitorum, extensor digiti minimi
Wrist adduction (medial/ulnar flexion)	Flexor carpi ulnaris, extensor carpi ulnaris
Wrist abduction (lateral/radial flexion)	Flexor carpi radialis, extensor carpi radialis longus, extensor carpi radialis brevis
Finger flexion	Flexor digitorum superficialis, flexor digitorum profundus
Finger extension	Extensor digitorum, extensor indicis, extensor digiti minimi
Finger adduction	Palmar interossei
Finger abduction	Dorsal interossei, abductor digiti minimi
Thumb flexion	Flexor pollicis longus, flexor pollicis brevis
Thumb extension	Extensor pollicis longus, extensor pollicis brevis, abductor pollicis longus
Thumb adduction	Adductor pollicis
Thumb abduction	Abductor pollicis longus, abductor pollicis brevis

between the metacarpals. The muscles of the thumb are abductor pollicis brevis, opponens pollicis, adductor pollicis, and flexor pollicis brevis, which variously abduct, adduct, and flex the thumb. Opponens pollicis also rotates the first metacarpal to bring the thumb in front of the palm facing the fingers, the opposed position that enables the hand to grip objects firmly between the thumb and fingers. The muscles of the little finger are the abductor digiti minimi, flexor digiti minimi brevis, and opponens digiti minimi. These muscles abduct and flex the little finger. The opponens digiti minimi also rotates the fifth metacarpal, so that the little finger faces the thumb; like the opposition of the thumb, this contributes to the ability of the hand to grasp effectively. The muscles of the palmar region are the lumbricals and the dorsal and palmar interossei, which flex the metacarpophalangeal joints (knuckles) and extend the interphalangeal joints of the fingers. The palmar interossei also adduct the fingers towards the middle finger and the dorsal interossei have the opposite function of abducting the fingers.

Hand injuries are relatively common in sports that require interaction with equipment, such as basketball. Many of these injuries are to bony structures, but traumatic injuries also include ligament ruptures in the digits; these injuries usually occur as a result of misjudging a catch. Hitting sports that involve the hand and wrist may put the wrist at risk of overuse injury from repeated movements under tension, particularly if the technique used is incorrect. For example, excessive tension and flexion of the wrist with the finger flexors activated can lead to carpal tunnel syndrome where the flexor tendons become inflamed through overuse. This is a potentially serious condition that may require surgical intervention. As with most overuse injuries, the root cause should be identified after recovery and rehabilitation from the injury to prevent recurrence once training is resumed. Errors in technique, or simply increasing training volume too quickly, are often causes of overuse injury, regardless of the specific sport involved.

See also: **muscle; wrist and hand; wrist and hand – bones; wrist and hand – joints; wrist and hand – ligaments.**

Bibliography

Bonanno, D. R., Landorf, K. B., Munteanu, S. E., Murley, G. S., & Menz, H. B. (2017). Effectiveness of foot orthoses and shock-absorbing insoles for the prevention of injury: A systematic review and meta-analysis. *British Journal of Sports Medicine, 51,* 86–96.

De Blaiser, C., Roosen, P., Willems, T., Danneels, L., Vanden Bossche, L., & De Ridder, R. (2017). Is core stability a risk factor for lower extremity injuries in an athletic population? A systematic review. *Physical Therapy in Sport, 30,* 48–56.

De Smedt, T., de Jong, A., Van Leemput, W., Lieven, D., & Van Glabbeek, F. (2007). Lateral epicondylitis in tennis: Update on aetiology, biomechanics and treatment. *British Journal of Sports Medicine, 41*(11), 816. doi: 10.1136/bjsm.2007.036723.

de Vries, J. S., Krips, R., Sierevelt, I.N., Blankevoort, L., & van Dijk, C. N. (2011). Interventions for treating chronic ankle instability. *Cochrane Database of Systematic Reviews*, 8. Art. No.: CD004124. DOI: 10.1002/14651858. CD004124.pub3.

Dines, J. S., Bedi, A., Williams, P. N., Dodson, C. C., Ellenbecker, T. S., Altchek, D. W., . . . Dines, D. M. (2015). Tennis injuries: Epidemiology, pathophysiology, and treatment. *Journal of the American Academy of Orthopedic Surgeons, 23,* 181–189.

Emery, C. A., Black, A. M., Kolstad, A., Martinez, G., Nettel-Aguirre, A., Engebretsen, L., . . . Schneider, K. (2017). What strategies can be used to effectively reduce the risk of concussion in sport? A systematic review. *British Journal of Sports Medicine, 51*(12), 978. doi: 10.1136/bjsports-2016-097452.

Evans, G., & Redgrave, A. (2016). Great Britain rowing team guideline for diagnosis and management of rib stress injury: Part 1. *British Journal of Sports Medicine, 50,* 266–269.

Evenson, K. R., Goto, M. M., & Furberg R. D. (2015). Systematic review of the validity and reliability of consumer-wearable activity trackers. *International Journal of Behavioral Nutrition and Physical Activity, 12,* 159.

Gribble, P. A., Bleakley, C. M., Caulfield, B. M., Docherty, C. L., Fourchet, F., Fong, D. T., . . . Delahunt, E. (2016). Evidence review for the 2016 international ankle consortium consensus statement on the prevalence, impact and long-term consequences of lateral ankle sprains. *British Journal of Sports Medicine, 50*(24), 1496. doi: 10.1136/bjsports-2016-096189.

Hall, J. P. L., Barton, C., Jones, P. R., & Morrissey, D. (2013). The biomechanical differences between barefoot and shod distance running: A systematic review and meta-analysis. *Sports Medicine, 43*, 1335–1353.

Hewett, T. E., Myer, G. D., Ford, K. R., Paterno, M. V., & Quatman, C. E. (2016). Mechanisms, prediction, and prevention of ACL injuries: Cut risk with three sharpened and validated tools. *Journal of Orthopaedic Research, 34*(11), 1843–1855. http://doi.org/10.1002/jor.23414

Kelikian, A. S. (Ed.) (2011). *Sarrafian's anatomy of the foot and ankle: Descriptive, topographic, functional* (3rd ed.). Philadelphia, PA: Lippincott Williams & Wilkins.

Knudson, D. V. (2013). *Qualitative diagnosis of human movement: Improving performance in sport and exercise* (3rd ed.). Champaign, IL: Human Kinetics.

Levine, D., Richards, J., & Whittle, M. W. (Eds.) (2012). *Whittle's gait analysis* (5th ed.). Oxford: Churchill Livingstone Elsevier.

Moore, K. L., Agur, A. M. R., & Dalley, A. F. (2011). *Essential clinical anatomy* (4th ed.). Philadelphia, PA: Lippincott Williams & Wilkins.

Morton, S., Barton, C. J., Rice, S., & Morrissey, D. (2014). Risk factors and successful interventions for cricket-related low back pain: A systematic review. *British Journal of Sports Medicine, 48*, 685–691.

O'Connor, K. L., Rowson, S., Duma, S. M., & Broglio, S. P. (2017). Head-impact-measurement devices: A systematic review. *Journal of Athletic Training, 52*(3), 206–227. doi: 10.4085/1062-6050.52.2.05.

Sewell, D., Watkins, P., & Griffin, M. (2013). *Sport and exercise science: An introduction* (2nd ed.). London: Routledge.

Struyf, F., Tate, A., Kuppens, K., Feijen, S., & Michener, L. A. (2017). Musculoskeletal dysfunctions associated with swimmers' shoulder. *British Journal of Sports Medicine, 51*, 775–780. doi: 10.1136/bjsports-2016-096847.

Warden, S. J., Davis, I. S. & Fredericson, M. (2014). Management and prevention of bone stress injuries in long-distance runners. *Journal of Orthopaedic and Sports Physical Therapy, 44*, 749–765.

Watkins, J. (2014). *Fundamental biomechanics of sport and exercise.* London: Routledge.

Wilson, F., Gissane, C., & McGregor, A. (2014). Ergometer training volume and previous injury predict back pain in rowing: Strategies for injury prevention and rehabilitation. *British Journal of Sports Medicine, 48*, 1534–1537.

Index

9780367150563